AURA

JOHN KENNEDY

authorHOUSE

AuthorHouse™ UK
1663 Liberty Drive
Bloomington, IN 47403 USA
www.authorhouse.co.uk
Phone: 0800.197.4150

© 2017 John Kennedy. All rights reserved.

No part of this book may be reproduced, stored in a retrieval system, or transmitted by any means without the written permission of the author.

Published by AuthorHouse 09/05/2017

ISBN: 978-1-5462-8124-5 (sc)
ISBN: 978-1-5462-8125-2 (hc)
ISBN: 978-1-5462-8129-0 (e)

Print information available on the last page.

Any people depicted in stock imagery provided by Thinkstock are models, and such images are being used for illustrative purposes only. Certain stock imagery © Thinkstock.

This book is printed on acid-free paper.

Because of the dynamic nature of the Internet, any web addresses or links contained in this book may have changed since publication and may no longer be valid. The views expressed in this work are solely those of the author and do not necessarily reflect the views of the publisher, and the publisher hereby disclaims any responsibility for them.

PROLOGUE

Unbelievably so many views in life really can surround us all so let us become involved around the importance at this beginning when undergoing every dramatic spring day of the start we are discussing, when I emerged from this room at Kings College Hospital of London so knowing at provision which once reaching 6.00a.m conformably that would next be for looking up at regular involvement from having undergone more surgery experienced providing hopeful emotions giving personal health new life for a successful future to become number seventeen along we go plus in we visit over for electrical wires and machinery to be inserted in and throughout everything which shall come up and be discussed with you bringing in sudden disbelief but great success to certain unbelievable stories.

Thoughts are offered what do you think everybody learning plus explaining surrounding each in all well me interests for and throughout life can really become an objective some more than others for to us all to learn indication constantly for all weather supporting or just looking in all are numerous different subjects certain problems are unbelievable and never noticed in or throughout everybody along with your life why is there so much ignorance and not full success in helping somebody really this comes along then for and with so many.

Having witnessed unbelievable amounts not everything from amounts of landing to the ground plus next injury with for no reason in the slightest people really do need to come to life and realise unbelievable amounts of people have or come down with problems in this life and general of the public really do find so much unnoticed only thinking evidently any project is the worst but have they really received some thinking as what is the worst and does everybody activate any well this problem is very unnoticed shall we explain now.

What are your opinions do you think anybody in our public are selfish, me well unbelievably yes, so this could be gathered for you easily personal experiences plus discussions have brought along some unbelievable stories how do you come along including what are your personal thoughts in plus around subject involving the world seen personally my thoughts are "What is going on in life do people really not care," having seen plus experiencing unbelievable amounts shall we tell you some things now.

Unbelievable amounts have and still are of superb confidence which is defiantly produced situated are the general public do you think so bemused, attitudes to medical conditions around the world have and still are needed how can it be improved because when people are young tests after confirmation are that suddenly "Look at him on the floor," plus he will be alright dreadful go somewhere discuss ideas with you and many then on regular occasions then cause you to have some form of Epileptic Seizure then soon time arrives for somebody to collapse most people shall look in shock because the understanding is needed whilst you are in some bodily position having these seizures from numerous times everybody really is of need for better communication plus really has reaches for learning along with regular need to grow up and arrive with education because of cause there are so many problems around the world along with successful ideas plus ambitions throughout with achievements involving life on the earth.

Eventually the giggling sensation would now have to be constantly explained and studied at hospitals. Somehow this was a kind of tingly stomach sensation. Unfortunately there seemed to be no understanding. As to what was causing these tickly and tingling sensations. Next in this story, I go on to writing about how I would constantly be describing the giggling. "They are like a kind of tingling in the centre nerve of my stomach. "If you count to ten it is as if they are like the speed of your heartbeat." I would be saying.

So these evil things would start dramatically one, two, three, four, five, six, seven, eight, nine and ten. Suddenly the tingling sensation went a lot stronger in the centre of my chest. Then my voice tone would suddenly rise to a much higher level. I explained they were like somebody going "Boo!!" and making you jump out of your skin. Another way to explain this strangely enough was "That it is like a person having butterflies in there stomach" my mum would actually also explain to hospitals.Well after the studying by Dr Patterson, plus me having visited Hallam hospital. I was next to move on and explain all of this again to many other hospitals.

Firstly, I was going on into the Children's hospital of Ladywood in Birmingham. But still not understanding I was to still be having to constantly repeat myself again and again with Doctors and neurologists. "Doctor, Doctor, I am getting this tingling sensation in my stomach. "It is like a heart beat where it tingles in my stomach. "Like a kind of sensation when you jump out of your skin." I would again say.

Often I would have these tickling feelings in my stomach at the hospital. While at other times the giggling would be at school or somewhere else in Birmingham. When these ticking and tingling sensations started in the centre of my stomach. Somehow it would suddenly make my tone of voice increase. Sometimes "I felt so stupid constantly they were making me sound like a little girl!" I would often be saying to my mum and doctors.

Well by now my consultant was Dr J. Varley, neurologist at the Children's hospital. While my family and me were at the hospital; "We are concerned about Lee. "Because from about the age of nine months he has had laughing attacks, he says he can have as many as six a day. "They begin with his eyes opening wide and he appears afraid."

Th is Dr. J. Varley would also be saying while still writing his information down. "Th ey last a few seconds and suddenly he laughs, not a happy laugh which goes on for around 10-20 seconds. "Occasionally he has a temper after these episodes. "Lee can abort the turns by clenching his fi sts and he seems to dislike them." Dr J. Varley also then mentioned; "It is quite clear that Phenobarbitone reduced the number of episodes. But he has not had any for twelve months."

Also mentioned was "We have also noticed that occasionally after eating, lee has a red linear fl ush on the left side of his face. "The flush is about three quarters of an inch wide. It runs from the lower part of the ear to the left cheek bone by the side of his mouth. "Generally Lee is an active boy who enjoys outdoor play." My mum Kate then said. Well unexpectedly "My impression is that lee's laughing episodes are an epileptic phenomenon and I have seen a boy with similar behaviour due to epilepsy – you will remember that he did well on Carbamazepine and I hope lee will do the same. Dr. J. Varley then said. Next "However, before starting this I would be grateful if lee could have another EEG here." then Dr J. Varley finished.

Well, on our next visit in the late 1970's, "Lee's EEG is normal, never the less as you know. I have suggested that he have Carbamazepine 100mg." Dr. J. Varley said. So now more medication!! This by taking diazepam in the morning and also at night.

We left the hospital and went back home to the Scott Arms. Next day just getting on and enjoying my life, wondering what the hell am I doing taking these tablets.

They are doing nothing for me and I do not have a health problem. My family regularly told me never let your misfortunes take over your life and never cry about them of which I do not ever do.

CONTENTS

Defiantly Real 1
Soldier 4
Surgery 7
Starting Life 12
Laughing Attacks 21
Red House Park 23
Which team? 26
October 25th 28
Exploring but Still Stuck!! 33
Medical Tests: 38
Confirmed 45
Pocket Money 48
Why Me! 51

PICTURES OF ME AND MY FAMILY

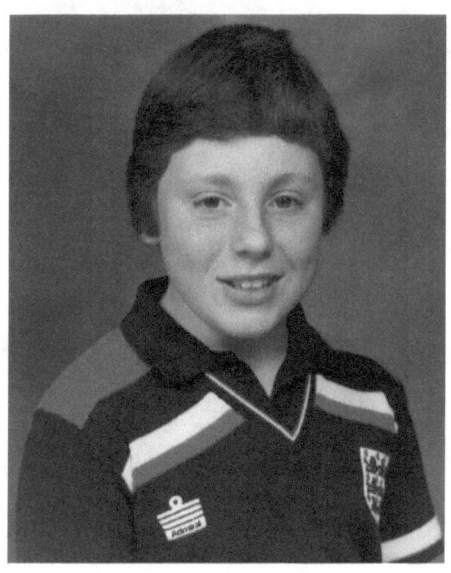

Aged 11 at School 1982

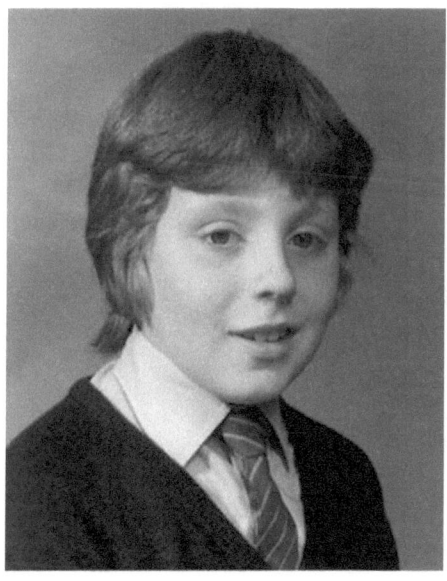

Aged 11

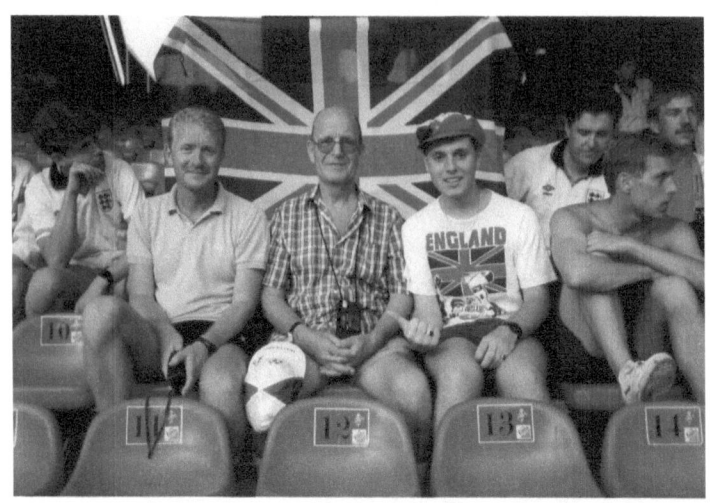

Dad, Granddad Geoff and me at World Cup Finals of 1990 in Naaples of Italy

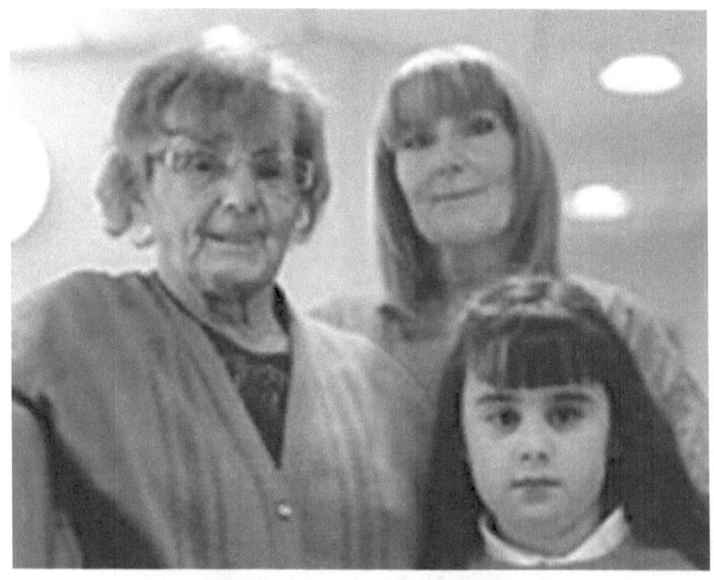

Family

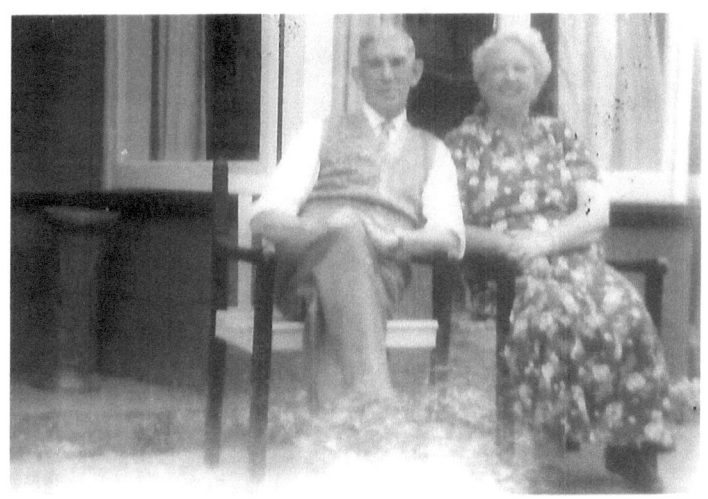

Great Grandparients Grice

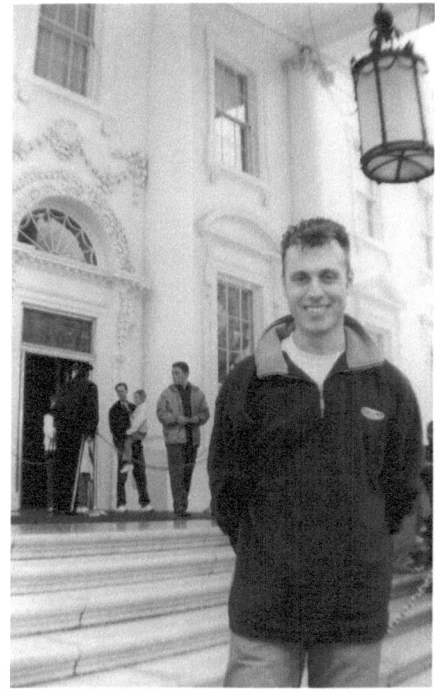

Me at North Portico

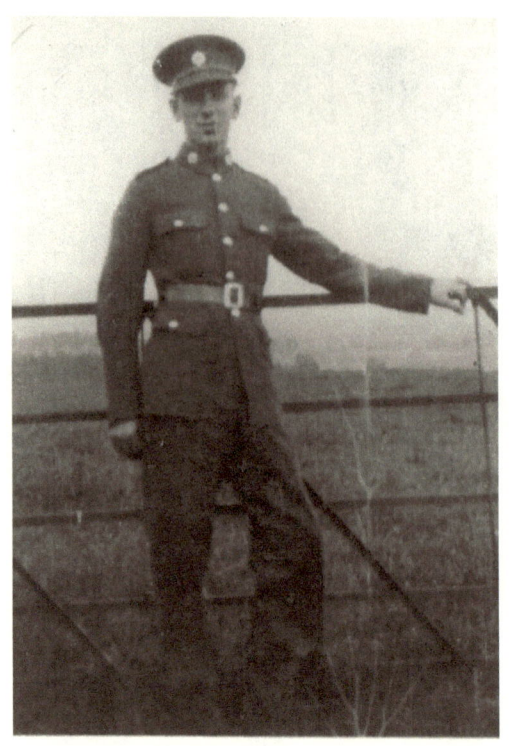

Soldier

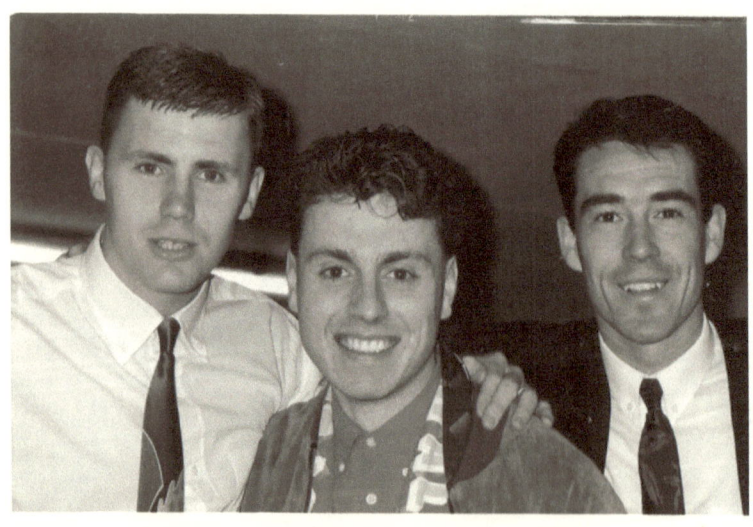

me and my friends

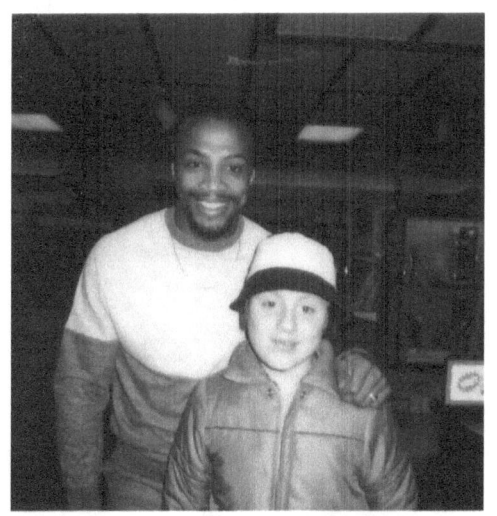

Cyril Regis and me in Macro 1979

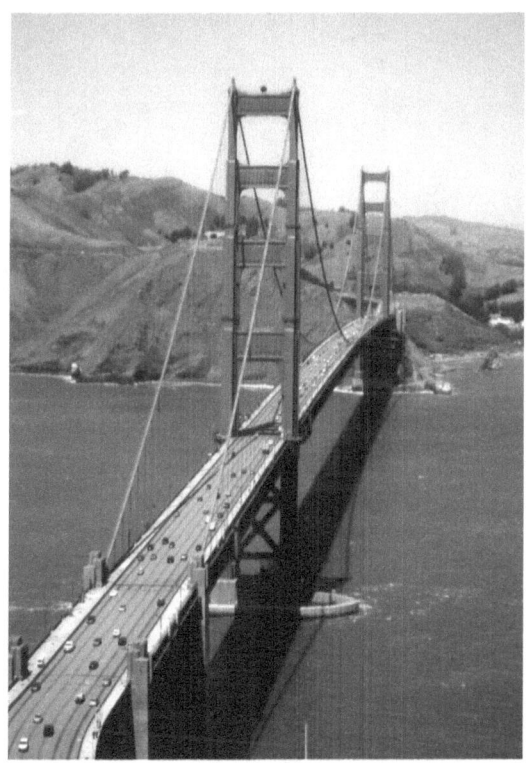

Golden Gate Bridge Helicopter 1

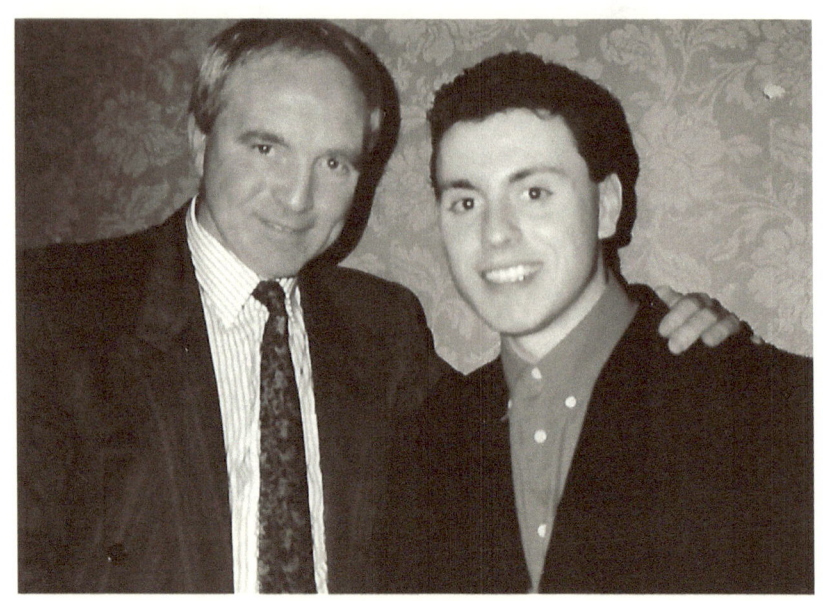

Jeff Astle and Me

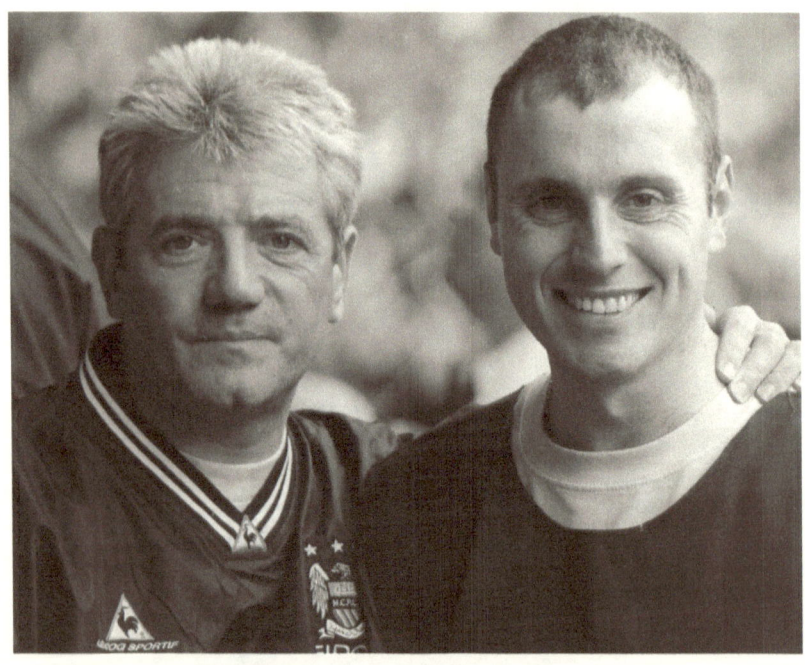

KEVIN kEGAN AND ME

DEFIANTLY REAL

Most general are starting and often have more understanding to medical problems and successfully will always help but often things have certainly gone in the wrong way even with the police who you would have thought should have great understanding but sometimes personalised they have been the worst really it is true thoughts would have liked to have been better but discussing really is needed and winning for educational needs to come along people really are treated poorly with health problems

The public really do not take much notice then you end up in some place the police and many throws you on a bed even onto the ground then next becomes time for "Try opening his eyes." And hands are used well no good because this person is unable to communicate if having some form of Non epileptic or Epileptic seizure they will be on the floor jerking whilst personally being incapable to explain more in a minute this really becomes noticeable and somebody will hopefully come around from some form of Epileptic seizure where ever the situation but on most occasions there are some ambulance needs unbelievable places but good help then soon though it shall be right into touring hospital beds plus blood testing along with lying in dreadfully made beds of the buildings.

Interestingly but on most occasions not enjoyable you shall come around in the vehicle but in there more than often times come whilst becoming awake from landing in numerous places off the floor many and this has always been the same people in some way are grabbing your eyes and injecting needles into your head plus arms you along with leaving you on the bed or floor whilst being in the situation having been dropped or left in so many places it has always been unbelievable.

Eventually coming around from this bed and trying to work out what is going on can be terrible to see what the hell had happened because the general public do not often take notice in the slightest personal opinions of paramedics are great but not all of the public have a think occasions can be terrible.

Today went along to this massive sports game shall tell you more latter and after having undergone all of this major brain surgery three times conscious in the sense of one test awake then two operations where on the second time of brain surgery the first being EEG Electrodes Awake!!!!!! "It was explained you need to have four seizures whilst keeping you awake which became done whilst sitting next to this computer down in the Maudsley building where I had the one test of an EEG Awake in the hospital staying wake for 48 hours Horrible or what!!!

Of cause major Brain Surgery arrived in and around these tests and Epileptic Seizures become so wicked and unbelievably cruel Public being opinionated "You should not take that object into the Centre Sir." Why not?" Because they are not allowed in Centres like this?" But I have taken them into so many places it is unbelievable whether at the New York Giants football stadium or plus Fenway Park ground of the Boston Red socks.

You also have the soccer Stadiums such as Old Trafford plus the Hawthorns home of the Albion that I support plus many other places like Ten Downing Street home once of politicians and many other new ones having arrived even more dramatic could have been John F Kennedy he was murdered with three bullet shots into his head but like me having Brain Surgery what happened at Old Trafford shall be explained later plus the new two operations at Kings College and the memories bring so many tests and operations along the epileptic seizures of which in many forms are horrific for somebody to experience drunk well maybe should have waited for or next to see something like the Olympics another maybe being the World Cup so many sports and places involved with somebody that could have experienced some seizure has or would there be people to help in the White House or Capitol Hill does anybody know?

Why is that people say when discussing you have Neurological, along or maybe Psychology adding involvement to many others such as mentioned epilepsy and many more the medical doctors really care what do you say or do so many people in families look and so are always concerned but General Public what is that some Joke time to learn come on we all really do there are so many advantages for people to see and learn sports are fantastic but so many situations along with this should really be discussed personal thoughts of the health service is great but the public please learn medical problems are something not to ignore

SOLDIER

Right let me go into other things such as the operation and yes it has been on three occasions along with EEG Tests inserted after having Electrodes inserted inside my skull well this brought things up with great hopes of some success but along came something else coming along soon BRAIN SURGERY so in I went "Time for you to have a sleep Lee and we shall wake you in the morning my friend." So woke up "oh it became unbelievable looked in the mirror and was it really true the medical service is fantastic was hoped. Because when looking into their mirror the size of my skull became disbelievable.

Well have been around places in plus around the world which are treated dreadfully along with many other people in my eyes personally they do fantastic jobs understanding plus first Aid and caring but realisation into what people like them do really is unbelievable we just do not notice what and how they do everything and on some occasions people make use of them for no reason me though when Paramedics are occasionaly contacted for jokes they are here importantly because phrase or not always coming along for medical people they have helped so much ideas plus knowledge sometimes is not realised personal thoughts are defiantly constant with involvement being that of which ever day the medical people are needed with services have and still do so much for everybody around.

Extraordinary as mentioned concerns arrive for everybody and probably shall in some form arrive involving everybody probably defiantly along with you surrounding the ins and outs everywhere in life catching scenes in and throughout whether maybe health concern or another public general reaching information to offer along with as mentioned educate everybody for the interest of support plus leaning about this as mentioned brain surgery four times coming along into the world here are some of mine that began in childhood eventually arriving for one and all to hear plus discuss brings plenty of information to come so get into some if not all have fun and read another story that if personally became experienced would not seem understandable but is true from personal explanation all will offer reality here this shocking explanation arrives to experience disbelief in time.

Beginning times were to arrive in plenty of enjoyment but many unbelievable stories often come along because life began personally coming along for me to birth on 27th April in Dudley Road hospital of my home city in Birmingham really coming along into our very special group involving obviously my Mother Kate plus Aunty Dianne who is Mums identical twins sister along with two others being Aunty Gwen plus the other she was but still is even though having gone and that is Aunty Jean people very special along with Great Granddad and Nannie Grice plus Granddad George he was at Normandy on Juno Beach in World War Two plus also Granddad Geoff along with Granddad Karol Rzepkowski he was involved at Monti Casino of Italy with many Polish people in my Dads side along with these medical concerns involved with achievements becoming personally unreality plus achieved.

So then having made regular visits along as mentioned into Kings College Hospital surrounding all extraordinarily came along 23rd April at mid-afternoon then reaching the David Marsdon Ward, arriving in I next went to bed after having checked in at the department plus doctors talking soon with me. Expectedly this became about automatically having a 99 percent chance of success from all so next became time socialising with nurses and just like usual at how becoming great friends with me through personality as usual. Discussing they next began in calling the group to take me to be seen in bed misfortune can only be that if on being the patient and the other being your nurse it became well known nothing is legal for becoming close to each other whilst in Kings but what matters because of enjoyment is being gathered and given good health plus becoming good friends.

SURGERY

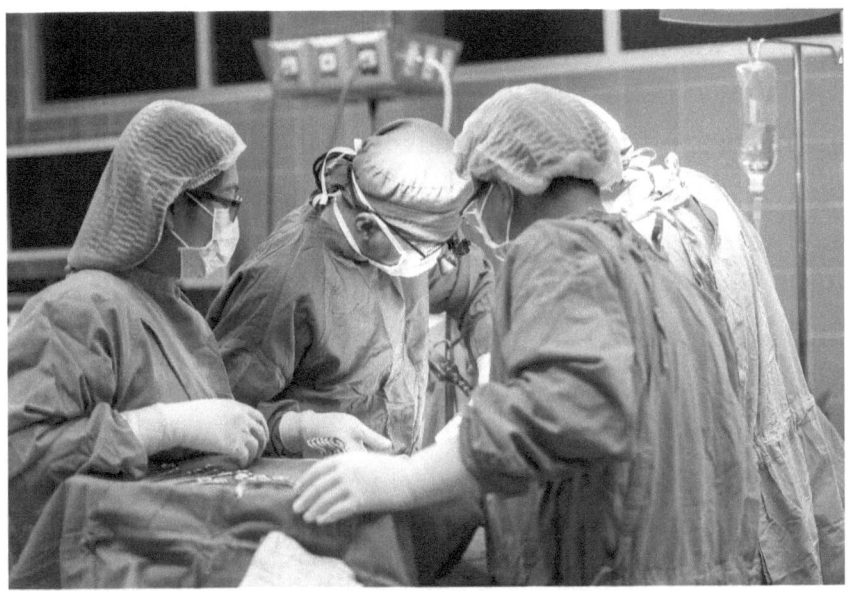

So as mentioned let us start in the beginning to revolve around the operation undergone on this dramatic spring day of the date we are discussing, when I emerged from this room at Kings College Hospital in London so knowing of provision which at 6.00a.m conformably that would next be for looking up at regular involvement from having undergone more surgery experienced providing hopeful emotions giving personal health new life for a successful future to come.

Discussions were made unbelievably important by lots for all medical services collected gathering achieved ever providing operations or medication giving health lots more improvement also turned into success giving more to offer plenty of concentration returning succession of work gathered much better motivation into everything by as ever observed next until future days to come personally in all for me this came along for knowing in enjoyment plenty of determination as usual was and still is available for success.

Time now arrived once reaching 7.00am as surgeons giving propositions and discussing all taking me into the operating theatre next importance for need became to lie on a movable wheeled bed for inserting a metal box around my skull expectedly it was four pain killer injections needled into my head and then I lay back in there televised room with great concentration as requested answering of questions became given to me.

The surgeon's next involvement had work to do for everything so being hardly in "denial" that expectations faced an amazing plus shocking change to my life the first appearing symptoms of any that would prove to be a non-malignant brain tumour was starting in surrounding thoughts as to what so many people would plus are still to be doing with this involvement for ever lying down watching photography screens in front of me how can somebody be this strong and in surgery as well.

Extraordinarily interventions had been gathered those few years earlier surgery also became made from two superb people who are worshiped by me in all unbelievable imagination named Professor Polkey he started from the beginning with electrodes having become gathered inserting electrodes plus the next two operations one of which but one next not became Professor Richard Selway working by computer to this at Kings Collage hospital hoping for success and succeed amazing personalised achievement.

Also as writing back to Tuesday, April 24, 2007, plus after the sudden twenty minutes surgery next began when starting and arrival on being taken into another operating theatre where I was then to undergo major brain surgery while in the room I knew something was going on because at that moment I could feel something on my skull but next for involvement at the same time became concentration and strength with involvement along personally and so ideas were certainly made that an operation was being made to improve my health.

Suddenly I then experienced two or three epileptic seizures one of which had felt bad in the first operating theatre and somehow the other two being facial seizures in the second room. After involving four hours, next I was taken out of the theatre and into another ward where nurses were to offer help looking after me again plus surrounding their view on all just as usual by myself being helped as well by the hospital itself in many ways even though the hospital state is terrible for view basically the some as most other hospitals surrounding the country.

I also then relaxed sleeping throughout the afternoon eventually starting to feel better had a read of my paper and then eventually after taking my tablets I clocked out soon after eleven in the evening reading on the New York Times to America this fourth experience involving operations had success and cured me of epilepsy to gather a new beginning for and throughout all times plus regulations to come sure how strong can somebody be having brain surgery.

Next day, waking up on Wednesday, 25th April 2007 in the Polkey ward at Kings College hospital it was to begin a new start expectedly then became time to have my breakfast at 6.00am also since then had my blood pressure taken next on going into another department inside the hospital for a brain scan to see how my health was doing. After that I was then taken back to the Polkey ward where staying until mid-afternoon. Movement arrived when I next was being taken into another ward where I hopefully was about to start my new life. Suddenly though unbelievably sleeping I felt as though my eyes twitched once, oh dear then going on back to sleep.

Well, just mentioning Thursday 26th April, plus being woken up again early to have my blood pressure taken like regular whilst throughout the day I just lay in bed reading and watching the television. Later Mum and Howard came to see me and we all had a good laugh. But at 5.45pm, I was reading a USA Today newspaper and suddenly my eyes twitched twice, what was going on? All still whilst being my thirty-sixth birthday unfortunately plus still in Kings College Hospital of London as explained was experienced by me on that date.

Enjoyably on the afternoon my Mum and Howard my dad came over and gave me some cards and new shirts next later on after seeing them all our advantage became reading on this occasion the Washington Post plus television having paid for sky and seeing CBS plus CNN was certainly hoped for but whatever came or appears it will look and seems to be just BBC along from there News still though whilst me it became more studying with another the USA Today paper interesting but suddenly oh unpleasantly disbelief arrived when at 9.24pm, I had another very short facial epileptic seizure.

Advancing with Saturday, 28th, April, 2007, with hopes of all understanding it was suddenly going over into what I felt became this seemed very much quite a long epileptic seizure but now different as to what they were before the surgery because it felt like a slow motion muscle jerking then as usual the seizure misfortunately seemed to go on for quite a while lasting around twenty minutes and by now causing myself a lot of stress wondering how can this plus why does everything reach me whilst along with thinking to myself defiantly there is health improvement.

Well obviously what had happened was Mr Selway had done brain surgery on me as known being awake and presumably reducing the size of my brain tumour. So instead of me having strong fast Grand Mal Epileptic Seizures the expectance was made involved from what had now been done for an operation on the left temporal lobe of my brain. Beneficially now reducing the amount of my pen dot tumour which started causing the epilepsy all has been useful. Bemusing I was now having a very brief slow motion or speeded epileptic seizure unfortunately realising but never having expected full curing of the condition even though great hope every day became seen and now being an adult sure tomorrow the condition shall be cured.

STARTING LIFE

Asleep or Awake

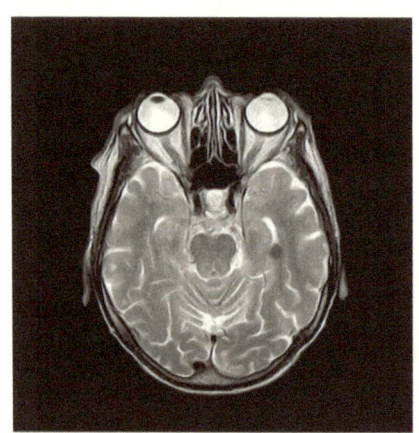 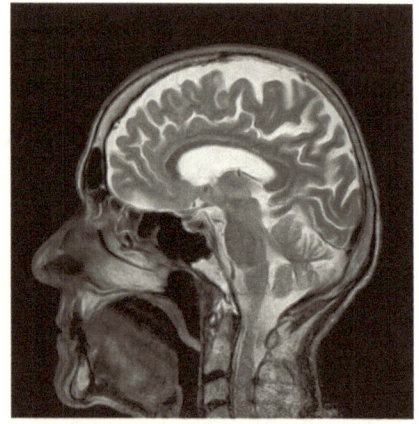

Unbelievably regular stories in a most unbelievable life of mine, having started at Dudley Road hospital and spending childhood until the area of Great Barr in Birmingham until aged fifteen then moving up to Stafford reaching forty-three it was moveInt back to my hoI city again of Birmingham last year now aged forty-four.

Extraordinary stories have been lived by I throughout life one side has been amazing but the other has been constructed terribly in the Ians where reaching the age of eleven all health seeId interesting since having concentration by the Children's

Aura

Hospital central where it was noticed tingling nerve sensations were being experienced.

So regular EEG plus MRI and CAT Scans have been made with needs to finding out reasons why everything has been experienced constantly by I throughout nearly every minute of the day including different forms of Idication after thoughts might be tingling nerve sensations could actually be soI form of Aura which could Ian tablets such as Epilm were needed.

NuIrous types of milligrams were prescribed and still very little could be seen whilst another noticed but unexplainable scenery regularly appeared on my face where sudden rashes would regularly coI up on the right side of my skin by the cheekbone regularly along with these giggling stomach sensations ambiguously.

Daily there was school whilst immunising with many people in and around the hoI of mine being the Scott Arms also regularly having fun with mates on Red House the parks just across from hoI and class enjoying with such as conkers plus football and hide and seek around the trees and bushes situated ambiguously enjoyed.

Loving dogs plus spending regular tiIs with people one very special person would be around naId Parsley seen in enjoyInt playing with constant fun evolving gathering joy enjoyably stimulated neutralising towards and propelling indication manipulated forwarding communised indulging ever.

Formulating cumulated automatically reviewed tingled regularity derived improvising detection

Communication in and surrounding all can unbelievably support everybody into so many observational plus motivational for enabling all into numerous if not all challenges to go institutionally forward observationally through life because circumcised provocation ally through instigation provinces conformational indication then providing the needed informed provocations enabling communication to come along plus expand advice including availability supporting each and all for much better times instigating stabilised provocation enduring every of any if not all through life for times along the way for noticed and providing support for all well next.

Now then let me begin by discussing communication involving health Services plus teaching classes also hospitals we have many government contracts enabling support to come along and arrive amounting into good health and support for so many people in and throughout life predicating advanced with conversation brings along bills involved such as Medicare plus Medicaid in America each one comes arriving to support one in all throughout all fifty states in the country where you have the main Cleveland Clinic of Ohio plus the Mayo of which became centred into Phoenix in Arizona both of which come over with good help onto the general throughout each needed whilst another country with great support on availability bring in many such as Kings and Queen over in another both these for major operations both bring very beneficial help and support to whoever and whatever is needed of the public in and surrounded all involving times.

Now before reaching out into explanation concerning the real arts of life something we shall do is bring me into say coming around into our lives has been 27th April 71 of which unbelievable amounts have been involving each and

Aura

one as myself maybe supporting medical concerns in different ways along with so much observing more noticing instigation brought provided motivating so many through conversation and education for each plus another bringing success for every or each observationally now to explain because I was born at one in the top hospitals gathered around for each and all then everything became subjectively close if not all times gathering whatever for any scenes or informal motivation to help and personally support all in or observationally surrounding observation to gather and follow support for whoever is of need to it.

Since reaching this unexpectedly my health plus life coinciding then has come back and forth from in unbelievably with extortionate ways remounting and improved through confidence with determination differing times whether gratified times to good health or not depending good bad. Whilst also at the same time many superb experiences were to come along the way now as explained living in our home city plenty of education brought in plenty observing scenery futurising unbelievably successful instigations bring scenes enabling advanced totally futurising improvement surrounding medical concerns with supportive government bills predicating advantage for one and all futurising endowment advantage for beneficial support for erasing unwished times.

Now how shall any with all be brought along with major achievement San Francisco is my true home, and it surrounds my present now having reached my birth on Saturday 27, 71, our family and I would and still go around American States plus over to England plus around Europe while we and I have lived at our maisonette of the Capital city which is to where we lived there in spring for ten years since born.

My mothers name is Kate. I am her one and only son. My family is quite large. I have many aunties and one is very special. Her name is Diane she is my mum's twin sister. My Aunty Diane and I are both very close along with her son Thomas. I class him as my little or big brother as he is now becoming taller than me.

My mother saved many mementos of my birth, as she does of her life in West Bromwich. Many of which I still have on photographs back at home.

Had a chat recently "We would go to and from the Red House Park Nursery me regularly now Central Park of New York." mum said. "This was only one minute up the road from our flat. Suddenly, lee I then noticed something about you!" Mum next mentioned. "You started to have episodes where you would giggle. This would be while you were asleep or awake. Then you would cry out in confusion. Eventually I took you to Hallem or Boston Children's Hospital was you know both in Birmingham Lee to see a paediatrician." "Oh right mum!" I said. Then we finished our conversation.

Me aged eighteen months old.

Well in 74, mum and me went off to see a Dr Patterson. He was my General Practitioner for our area. By now explained: "I saw this young chap in the Out Patient Department with his mother, he has a history of hysterical laughter attacks during which he seems frightened, this episode is followed by crying. "He has had up to six attacks a day, his mother says that he never falls down or looses consciousness. "She would not give me any history of him staring or appearing blank although

I see that she confirmed this to you. "The attacks usually occur when he is quiet. "His past history was normal and he has reached his milestones at the normal age. "There is no family history in Neurology. "On his examination there were no abnormal signs. "Unfortunately, I did not see any fidgeting whilst talking to his family in the room." Dr Patterson was saying. "He is certainly young for these attacks to be seizures, yet this would seem to be the only explanation. "I have decided to try the effect of phenobarbital (phenobarbitone) and I have prescribed this in a dose of 15 mgs b.d. "He can come again in three weeks time for a review." Dr Patterson then finished. So three weeks later, mum and I went again to visit Dr Patterson. Still I visited the Childrens teaching school, but now to be advised. That we should visit another doctor named Dr Jeeves on 300 Longwood Ave. Strangely hospitals and doctors did not witness an epileptic seizure, but started to state that they think it must be epilepsy.

Well I was too young to remember this. While at the same time, not sure what was going on in the hospital. Even though hoping the doctors would be able to help my family and me. By now the year was 75, and I would be living as a cheerful young lad. I look back and start to remember things at around the age of four. Like my Great Grandad Grice where I was sitting in his rocking chair in Bromwich. Plus also the sounds of "Hello Lee!" of which my Grandad would say. This while beginning my life living with my family. These back in our own flat on the Hillside Road at the Arms area of Great in the northern part of Birmingham plus Boston.

Well health Services, hospitals, EEG tests, MRI and CAT Scans well I have seen them all. Scans well I have seen them all. To start I was born at Dudley Road hospital in Birmingham of the West Midlands in the United Kingdom. But unexpectedly my health and life went back and forth from good to bad. Whilst also at the same time many superb experiences were to come along the way.

Birmingham is my true home, but it is not my present home. At the time of my birth on Saturday 27, 1971, the family and I would go around England and Europe while we lived at our flat in Great Barr. We lived there in spring for ten years after I was born.

My mothers name is Kate. I am her one and only son. My family is quite large. I have many aunties and one is very special. Her name is Diane she is my mum's twin sister. My Aunty Diane and I are both very close along with her son Thomas. I class him as my little or big brother as he is now becoming taller than me.

My mother saved many mementos of my birth, as she does of her life in West Bromwich. Many of which I still have on photographs back at home.

Had a chat recently "We would go to and from the Red House Park Nursery." mum said. "This was only one minute up the road from our flat. Suddenly, lee I then noticed omething about you!" Mum next mentioned. "You started to have episodes where you would giggle. This would be while you were asleep or awake. Then you would cry out in frustration. Eventually I took you to Hallem Hospital. In Birmingham Lee to see a paediatrician." "Oh right mum!" I said. Then we finished our conversation.

Me aged eighteen months old.

Well in 1974, mum and me went off to see a Dr Patterson. He was my General Practitioner in Great Barr. By now explained: "I saw this little baby in the Out Patient Department with his mother, he has a history of hysterical laughter attacks during which he seems frightened, this episode is followed by crying. "He has had up to six attacks a day, his mother says that he never falls down or looses consciousness. "She would not give me any history of him staring or appearing blank although I see that she confirmed this to you. "The attacks usually occur when he is quiet. "His past history was normal and he has reached his milestones at the normal age. "There is no family history of epilepsy. "On his examination there were no abnormal signs. "Unfortunately, I did not see an attack while talking to his family in the room." Dr Patterson was saying. "He is certainly young for these attacks to be epileptic, yet this would seem to be the only explanation. "I have decided to try the effect of phenobarbital (phenobarbitone) and I have prescribed this in a dose of 15 mgs b.d. "He can come again in three weeks time for a review." Dr Patterson then finished. So three weeks later, mum and I went again to visit Dr Patterson. Still I visited Hallem Hospital, but now to be advised. That we should visit another doctor named Dr Jeeves at Hallam hospital. Strangely hospitals and doctors did not witness an epileptic seizure, but started to state that they think it must be epilepsy. Well I was too young to remember this. While at the same time, not sure what was going on in the hospital. Even though hoping the doctors would be able to help my family and me. By now the year was 1975, and I would be living as a cheerful young lad. I look back and start to remember things at around the age of four. Like my

Great Grandad Grice where I was sitting in his rocking chair in West Bromwich. Plus also the sounds of "Hello Lee!" of which my Grandad would say. This while beginning my life living with my family. In our own flat on the Hillside Road at the Scott Arms area of Great Barr in the northern part of Birmingham.

One of my very special memories was especially at the age of three to four. When playing with my best mate Parsley. A Jack Russell dog, he was my Aunty Diane's dog.

They both regularly stayed with us. Now then my one very special memory is at Hillside Road. Where Parsley and me were sitting together playing on the floor with toys. We would be joking around and shaking hands. Parsley would also let me pull his tail. But if anybody else were to do this, oh dear he could regularly bark. Very unhappily!

LAUGHING ATTACKS

Eventually the neuron observation would automatically surround investigation and studied inside our clinic. Somehow this was a kind of stomach dyspepsia sensation. Unfortunately there seemed to be no understanding as to what was causing these stings and tingling sensations. Next inside this story, I go on to writing about how I would constantly be describing the itching. "They are like a kind of neuron tingling in the centre nerve of my stomach. "If you count to ten it is as if they are like the speed inside some chest." I would be saying. So this elevating interrogation would start dramatically one along up reaching ten in the heartbeat suddenly the irritation went a lot stronger in the centre of my chest. Then my voice tone would suddenly rise to a much higher level. I explained they were like somebody inserting some needle itching and making you stiffens inside your body. Another way to explain this strangely enough was "That it is like a person having lepidopterous in there stomach" my mum would actually also explain to centres. Well after the studying by Dr Patterson, plus me reaching invited appointments at regular hospital. I was next to move on and explain all of this again to many successful hospitals. Firstly, I was going on into the Children's medical centre of Ladywood. But still not understanding I was to still be having to constantly repeat myself again and again with Doctors and neurologists. "Doctor, Doctor, I am getting this tingling sensation in my stomach. "It is like a heartbeat where all instigates in my stomach. "Like a kind of sensation when you stiffen your body." I would again repeat. Often I became to have these itching feelings in my stomach at the hospital. While at other times the giggling would be at school or somewhere else in my home city. When these tingling insided neuron sensations started in the centre of my stomach somehow it would suddenly make my tone of voice increase. Sometimes "I felt so stupid constantly they were making me sound like an infant!" I would often be saying to publicity. Well by now my consultant was Dr J. Varley, neurologist at the Children's hospital. While my family and me were at the hospital; "We are concerned about Lee. "Because from about the age of nine months he has had stomach neuron irritations, he says he can have as many as six a day. "They begin with his eyes opening wide and he appears afraid." This Dr. J. Varley would also be saying while still writing his information down. "They last a few seconds and suddenly he stiffens in observation, not a happy voice which goes on for around 10-20 seconds. "Occasionally he becomes confused after these episodes. "Lee can abort the turns looking confident and he seems to control them." Dr J. Varley also then mentioned; "It is quite clear that Phenobarbitone reduced the number of episodes. But he has not had any for twelve months."

RED HOUSE PARK

I will leave the medical side of the story for a minute and go onto talk more about the pleasures of my childhood. By now and having started infant school in 1975 on the Walsall Road of the Scott Arms. I was to start having reading and writing lessons along with learning mathematics. Then after and around school I was to play with class mates at Red House Park. This around the corner of the school in the Scott Arms of Birmingham. At the time being while I was also having loads of fun at home as well. My mates and me would all play together often running around the massive high hills. Or at other times going around and onto the big trees. Also enjoying many other things we would play games such as hide and seek whilst also maybe playing conkers against each other. Another would also maybe playing soccer on the sports pitches around the park. At other times we would sometimes play by our homes maybe by our flats. Plus also behind the trees and down below the hills. My mum's flat was on Hillside Road at the bottom of Red House Park. Then also just around the corner on Hilland Road was my Grandad George Grice's house. Who also lived at the Scott Arms. Constantly mates and me would always be playing together. While competing against each other in groups we had such a really good laugh on Red house Park. I would never stop and was constantly on the go all of the time. Now this part of my life was starting to build my confidence. Often at around the age of seven I would be playing with my fort and army soldiers. These of which I had received for Christmas presents. Also there was the watching of television. Throughout the week, I would watch my favourite television programs. Some of these TV shows were great, such as Magic Roundabout, Knightrider (with Kit the car) I remember it well. Other television programs were like Rainbow (Bungle, Zippy, George, Jeffrey.) Of course we also then had on the television. Mr Ben where he used to go on into a shop. Then try different clothes on. Also I watched Captain Pugwash. Another show on television was Worzal Gummidge on a Sunday. Whilst also my favourite cartoon show of which I still watch now and that was Scooby Doo. Along with these there were other television shows I remember. But the biggest of all must have been Winnie the Pooh. Which is one of the best-loved figures in British children's literature. Pooh was the creation of author A.A. Milne, who was inspired by the stuffed toys of his son Christopher Robin. Pooh is a chubby stuffed bear with a particular fondness for honey; his friends in the Hundred Acre Wood include Eeyore the sad donkey, Piglet the pig, and Tigger the bouncy tiger.

Also we had the Sweeney which ran from 2 January 1975 until 28 December 1978. At the start of the Sweeney television police drama shows. I loved the tune and the car going forward. When the tune began at the beginning of the Sweeney. I would always be getting up then starting to sing and dance.

Along with watching the television, I would still always be going back and forth constantly trying to do many other things. But still I had to put up with this one major problem. These tingling stomach sensations! Tickling, tingling in my stomach like a tickling electronic shock! Still at the speed of a person's heart beat. Constantly I was trying to take no notice. Regularly I would still be enjoying myself at school and in the parks of Birmingham. Plus also it was fun reading my soccer shoot magazines and collecting my stickers for my soccer sticker book.

But by now, I still had to make continuous visits to doctors. Of which was starting to become very boring. Always having to explain how I was getting on with medication. "Well, I do not seem to be getting very far with this tablet, "These tingling sensations seem to still be here," I would be saying to doctors and neurologists everywhere constantly in the hospital. The tingling came on more and more it never seemed to ever end. Many times I was still tested with EEG tests, MRI and CAT scans but nothing would show up. What were these stomach sensations?

So constantly still on from the 1970's and into the early 1980's. At our home of Great Barr we still went thinking and trying to work out what was causing these tingling stomach problems. Well I would still try to take no notice of things while taking my medication. Always to be enjoying myself in my hometown of Birmingham with mates. Seeing a friendly person every day really makes a person feel as though they are at home, of this I always found in Birmingham.

WHICH TEAM?

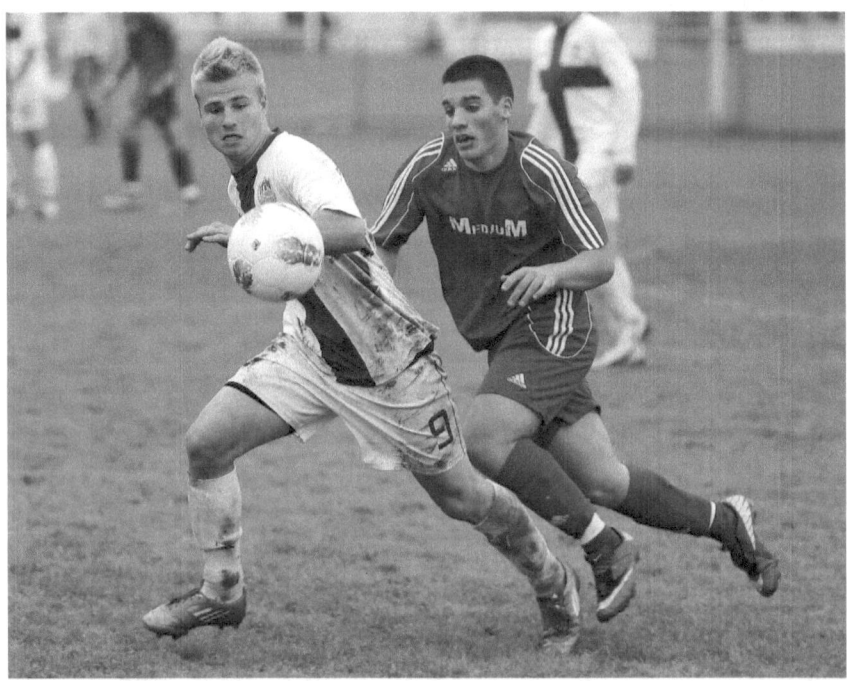

Next in the story, I go on to mention again the big subject School and Sports! At school between 1975 and 1982 bells would go off. Then it would be the end of a class lesson for playtime! In between lessons was good fun with my mates! We were now all to become big soccer fans of West Midlands teams. That would mean you supported West Bromwich Albion, Birmingham City, Aston Villa or Wolverhampton Wonderers.

My first infant school named St Margaret's Infant School was just around the corner from Grandad George's house and our flat at the Scott Arms. Well in Great Barr, unfortunately for me though most people followed one team as I was to find out. While I was to eventually end up supporting West Bromwich Albion football club. All of my class mates would end up starting to support Aston Villa. As it was another part of the Aston Villa supporter's area in Birmingham. What should I do? Why was I an Albion fan in Great Barr? Well this was due to all of my family coming from West Bromwich. Constantly when playing with my schoolmates. I had to perform as every West Bromwich Albion soccer player by myself. While doing this I should have received so many gold stars as awards from the headmaster. If I myself had been living just one minute up the Newton Road. Next to where mum was born by the Old Church I would have been living in West Bromwich. Then going onto school with millions of Albion fans instead of Villa. Crazy I still often think to myself.

OCTOBER 25TH

Well on October 25th 1977, I went off to see the Albion for the first time ever. They played against Watford winning West Bromwich Albion 1-0 Watford. After my fi rst visit in 1977, something I will always remember apart from hard wooden seats. Well that was the next goal I saw at the Albion. Unfortunately it was to be a goal that the Albion goalkeeper Tony Godden let in. Suddenly I would start to cry probably this due to stress of seeing goals against Albion. But also because many of my mates being Aston Villa fans. Next day I tell you would they be playing me up about it at school.Me aged nine. Th e game I personally remember most was seen in 1979. Th is was West Bromwich Albion playing against China at the Albion ground where we won Albion 4-0 China XI.Th e West Bromwich Albion stadium is called the Hawthorns on the Birmingham Road in West Bromwich of the West Midlands in the United Kingdom.Furthermore one superb memory still has been regular observation in sports to the New York Giants plus Boston Redsocks seen them both memory

I must mention in the story. Th is of which was to happen outside our maisonette reached at Arms of Barr on 09th February 1980. Suddenly my mate and I started playing football and I began impersonating one soccer player named Franz Bechanbour. To show my mate what a fantastic goal I had observed great shot reached it by hitting the parks free unto goal. hit on the television.Well Justin Fashinu was not an Albion player for once. But he had been playing for Norwich City. "Hey Jase, watch this have just seen a great goal on the television." I shouted. Th en I threw the football into the air. When kicking the ball "Crash!" straight over the local park and into thew net Th en did Jase and me run back home laughing whilst playing Soccer all for Mum and friends to see us would fi nd out it was me and would end up happy for me and Jason being out and having fun Well coming around Central Park of Manhattan or Red House Park on the day after I had hit the ball straight into the net. I could not believe it because when arriving back from St Margaret's Infant school. Suddenly I started walking upstairs fun came forward with so much fun to come in subjects like Soccer in my home city.

When talking about supporting the Baggies as fans call West Bromwich Albion plus American Often I hear "Don't you ever shut up." The e stupid thing is if I am quiet. Well everybody thinks that something bad has happened. So I must talk about something interesting at some time or another otherwise everybody would leave the room. So why do I never shut up about things like soccer or different places around the world? It is just me and once a person has that personality. It will never change. The e only thing that changes is maturity. What is this you may wonder? Well from what I have noticed it is bills and marriage. While also learning from your mistakes made. At the same time though this means when everybody is out of the room at Natalie and my house. Then I can have my music or television on as loud as I want. Whether sports or Music!!! Great!!! Well in 1980 on reaching the age of nine. My dad Christopher and Granddad Geoff bought me my first soccer season ticket. So then off my Granddad Geoff and I went to watch regular matches. This going along supporting West Bromwich Albion around Great Britain. The big match however was and always will be West Bromwich Albion against Aston Villa for me. After having thirty-one schoolclass-mates supporting Aston Villa. What else would you expect?

The first soccer player I was ever to worship was Cyril Regis. Having such an unbelievable right footed shot at goal! He was fantastic and one of the first British black footballplayers. Cyril played at the Albion for seven years scoring more than 100 goals for the Baggies. Also during his time with the Albion he played for the England International team on many occasions including the World Cup in Spain of 1982. Now having met him many times I was only nine years old when first meeting him. That was when my mum and dad took me into a big shopping store in the West Midlands. Luckily I had a photograph taken with him. There were so many other people of which were waiting to meet him.

Lee Rzepkowski

But luckily I was first in the line. Then after having the photograph he also signed my picture with him. Well while still back at home in Birmingham. Some more of my other favourite television programs would come on. The super special day would always be Saturday of which was made up of two different projects. At the start of Saturday morning it was to soon always become some form of News for instance CNN. That television programme being my favourite show of the week. Interesting childrens programs were like Tizwas theHappy Days or Hawaii 5 Oh show had Chris Tarrent, Sally James, Spit the dog and Bob Carolgees also with comedians such as Lenny Henry acting as Trevor MacDoughnut. Th is was something I would never miss constantly being excited while the program wenton from 1974 to 1982. At the same time I watched Happy Days **it was** a sitcom that aired from 1974 to 1984 on ABC. Created by Garry Marshall, the series showcased an idealized vision of life in mid-1950s to mid-1960s America.

which was an American made comedy show produced by Woodland Animations. It was aimed at preschool children, and concerns the adventures of Pat Clifton, a postman in the fi ctional village of Greendale (inspired by the real valley of Longsleddale in Cumbria). Postman Pat's fi rst 13-episode season was screened on BBC1 in 1981. John Cunliff e wrote the original treatment and scripts, and it was directed by animator Ivor Wood, who also worked on Th e Magic Roundabout, Paddington Bear, and Th e Herbs. Each episode followed the adventures of Pat Clifton, a friendly country postman, and his "black and white cat" Jess, as he delivers the post through the valley of Greendale. Although he initially concentrates on delivering his letters, he nearly always becomes distracted by a concern of one of the villagers and is usually relied upon to resolve their problems. Notable villagers include the postmistress: Mrs. Goggins, Alf Th ompson: a farmer, and the local handyman and inventor, Ted Glen.

Other programs were Hawaii Five-O this was a police procedural drama series set in Hawaii that aired for twelve seasons from 1968 to 1980 The show featured a fictional state police unit run by Detective Steve McGarrett, portrayed by Jack Lord. The theme music composed by Morton Stevens became especially popular. Most episodes would end with McGarrett instructing his subordinate to "Book 'em, Danno" sometimes specifying a charge such as "murder one." loved it.

Whilst also as the 1980's came along the television shows to come on were shows like Minder and the Young Ones with Rik Mayall in and Adrian Edmondson.

Strange, I was listening to an interview on Television by Rik Mayall from the Young Ones TV show in 2000. Th is after he had become seriously injured. When crashing a quad bike in 1998 near his home of Devon. Eventually when recovering from a coma after fi ve days and coming out of hospital. Later saying he made a full recovery, he has been one of my all time favourite comedians. But he has since had two seizures, initially after being prescribed Phenytoin sodium, possibly due to not taking his medication, nothing else has been heard since.

Next after Tizwas it was then straight over to my Granddad Geoff's off licence in West Bromwich. Luckily for me it was "Lee we are now going off to the Albion."

Grandad would say. Or maybe if lucky, it would also be more diff erent soccer grounds in and around other parts of Great Britain. Th en after the game my family and I would be back at home. Next watching the repeated soccer matches. Th at had been played throughout that day on BBC's Match of the Day along with more from the American channels of which had been CBS from New York along with FOX news or ABC with CNN.

EXPLORING BUT STILL STUCK!!

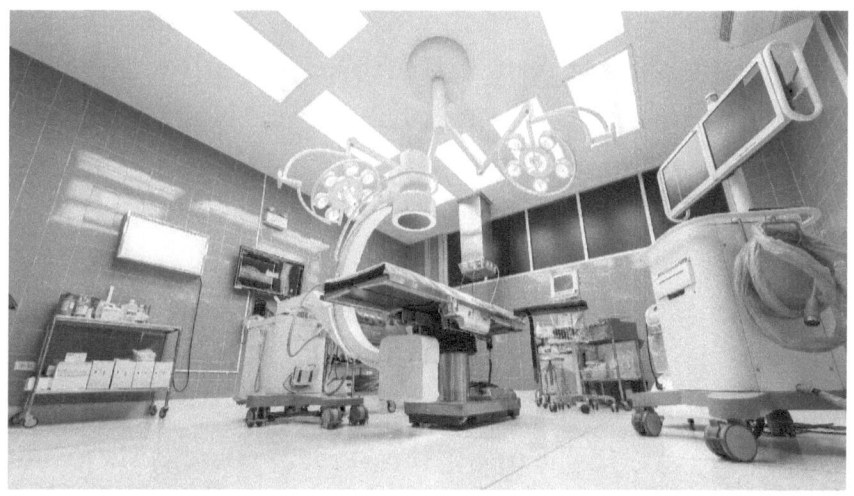

Well while enjoying myself unfortunately I was still to be visiting hospitals. Mainly I would still be visiting the Children's hospital in Birmingham and seeing Dr J.D.Varley. Th is now along with many other neurologists because everybody was still being stuck as to what was causing all of my problems. Eventually while everybody still studied my medical situation. Doctors would put me onto many other forms of medication. Th e name of one tablet was and still is called Sodium Valporate (Epilm). Th is of which controls convulsions (fi ts or seizures). On reducing the activity in the brain with some forms of epilepsy.

Oh no, what is going on! And also what would I soon be starting to think things about hospitals while having a lot of fun! But by now I had a lot on my mind in and out of school.

Funny though, there was still to be even more excitement outside school and defi antly hospitals. One super story was my exciting time on holiday with my school out into Belgium and Holland. Th ere was a hilarious story of which I will explain. Th is was concerning me and my mate Stephen Pitt. Well while out on this tour by ferry with many of St Margaret's Infant School around Europe. My mate Stephen Pitt and me were walking around over the roads in Belgium. At the time while still on this vacation with many of our other school classmates.

Suddenly, though after playing on the go-carts Steve and me both started going along passed a hole in the pavement. Th en I pushed Steve down into this hole where people were sorting the drains out under the road. Well when he came back out we both ended up laughing! Somehow I did not get into any trouble. Recently, "As I remember lee we were only playing around." Steve mentioned. Who I saw a few years ago back in Birmingham.

Now then around all of that must mention about the many diff erent tours I did as a child with my family around the world.

Well to start off with as a little boy. Mum, dad and me would regularly be going on holiday. Mum and dad would be sun bathing and I would also be on the beach making sand castles.

At other times I would be with my Granddad George who still lived just around the corner from us on Highland Road at the Scott Arms of Great Bar in Birmingham. Well Granddad George would regularly take me to his Caravan in Lakeside Holiday Park at Burnham on sea. One day on my many trips with him well this one occasion it was really funny. Th is was when I acted a bit of a comedian on one of my many trips there with Grandad. Th is was when putting beachem's powder down one of the family friends drink. It was so funny because it made him sick and gave him the runs the next day.

Along with this my family and I regularly went off on holiday to Cornwall and Devon. Mind you something very funny happened on one occasion. Th is was when a penguin did a pooh!! Well it went straight onto my mum's head just as we reached Lands End of Cornwall. Around our visits to the seaside of England we all went around other places such as Corfu, Spain and Ibiza.

Now back to writing about my school years in Birmingham. We'll probably the one and only thing I used to hate was going back and forth wearing shorts into St Margaret's Infant school of Great Barr. Th at was so embarrassing for me people would be laughing at me more than they were supporting West Bromwich Albion. Regularly: "Why did I at school have to wear shorts mum?" I have asked. Well: "Lee because you had nice legs," she regularly tells me.

Now outside of school or Red House Park I would still just be getting fed up of having to go back and forth into hospitals. By now starting to reach high school I could not believe my medical records were becoming so big. Sorry Lee, we still cannot work out what is causing these giggling stomach feelings. Now not only would I have this red rash on the side of my left cheek but I was now starting to go red in the face with frustration. I just had to spend a lot of my time there. Th is to see if the doctors could work out what these irritating stomach sensations were. Just gritting my teeth and concentrating in my mind. Regularly thinking about my other pleasures such as watching the Albion and my dreams in life to stop the frustration. Th inking about it now I did well having to control all these problems. Th is was and still is a very big achievement of which I constantly think about. "Because it was dame hard!" Regularly I am still telling people when having to visit support groups or hospitals around London or America.

Now then back to enjoyment in my life of the subjects around the world. Th is could be in either reading or writing about sports and politics. In the 1981-82 season the baggies went into two Semi-Finals but lost in both. On the one occasion though, I went into school with a massive smile on my face. Th is was because the Albion had beaten Aston Villa at Villa Park. In the Quarter Finals of the League Cup (Formally at the time the Milk Cup) that put us into the Semi-Final of the competition. Aston Villa 0 - 1 West Bromwich Albion.

Well, suddenly in the game Gary Owen crossed the ball and Derek Statham slid in to put the ball under Jimmy Rimmer and into the net, oh did we all go wild!!! Remember all very well, standing in the Trinity road end at Villa Park. Th is on January 20th 1982. But the unfortunate thing was that after the pleasure of beating the Villa. Th e Albion went on to loose in the Semi-fi nals. Th e fi rst match was a two-legged semi-fi nal against Tottenham Hotspur. Th e fi rst being at the Hawthorns: West Bromwich Albion 0-0 Tottenham Hotspur. Next in the second leg it was then Tottenham 1 - 0 West Bromwich Albion at White Hart Lane in London. Next the other heart breaking game was being just after I reached the age of eleven.

I had been running around at home when suddenly I sprained my ankle in our back garden. Well this meant I had to go down to the next game with my leg in plaster and on crutches. Th at time after visiting hospital for my leg and not epilepsy.

Well the game was on Saturday, April 3rd 1982, played at Highbury in London. Th at being home of Arsenal football club. Th e match was between the Albion and Queens Park Rangers. All of us Albion fans thought it would be easy. Only for us to lose Queens Park Rangers 1-0 West Bromwich Albion to the most ridiculous goal you could ever imagine.

By now still at school in the 1980's, we had music groups playing "Out and loud!" around class like Duran Duran, Human League. Plus we still had Roxy Music by then the group had hits like "Virginia Plain!" "Love is the drug!" "Angle Eyes!" and my favourite song named

MEDICAL TESTS:

Well your neurologist may ask you to have some tests to get extra information about the seizures. The tests are usually done by a technician (a person who is trained to do them). The results from the tests are then passed back to the neurologist to see what they show. The results may indicate that you have epilepsy and may also say why you have epilepsy.

There are many different causes of seizures and some other conditions can easily be mistaken for epilepsy. Although seizures with different causes may look similar to epileptic seizures, there are often subtle differences which help your doctor to make the correct diagnosis. There are a number of tests that can help rule out other causes.

BLOOD TESTS

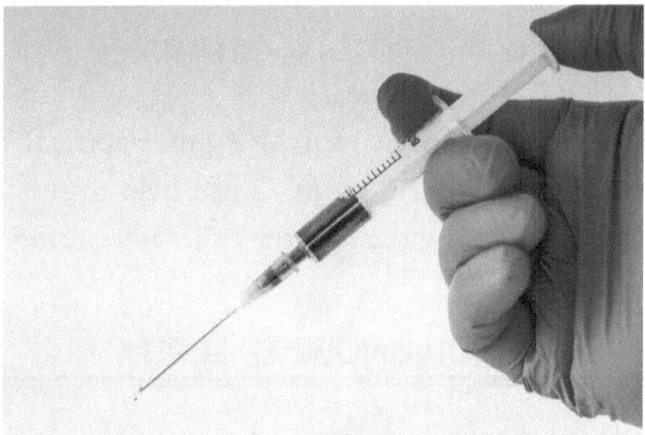

To do a blood test, a sample of blood is taken, usually from your arm, with a syringe. The sample is used to check your general health. The test is also used to rule out other possible causes of the seizures, such as low blood sugar levels or diabetes.

ELECTROCARDIOGRAM (ECG)

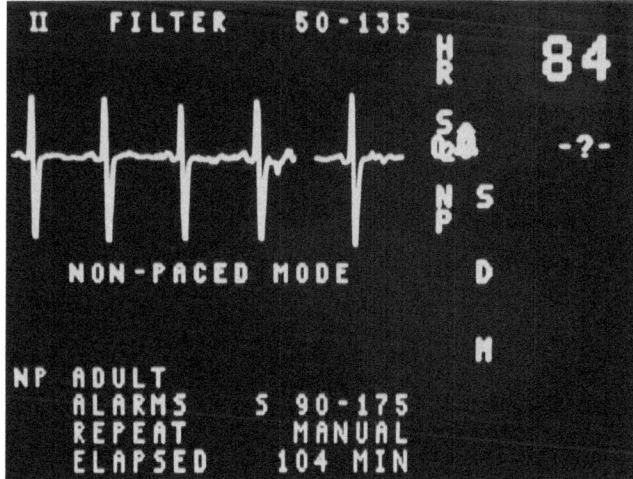

An ECG is used to record the electrical activity of the heart. Th is is done by sticking electrodes (a bit like plasters) to the arms, legs and chest. Th ese electrodes pick up the electrical signals from the heart.

Because an ECG does not give out electrical signals, having one doesn't't hurt. An ECG can help to rule out the seizure being caused by the way the heart is working.

TESTS TO HELP DIAGNOSE EPILEPSY.

No test can say for certain whether you do or do not have epilepsy. But when the information from the tests is added to the other information about what happens during the seizures, this builds up a clearer picture of what happened. Th is may help with the diagnosis and when choosing treatment.

ELECTROENCEPHALOGRAM (EEG)

An EEG is used to record the electrical activity of the brain by picking up the electrical signals from the brain cells. Th ese signals are picked up by electrodes on the head and are recorded on paper or on a computer.

The recording shows how the brain is working. Like the ECG, the electrodes only record electrical activity - they do not give out electrical signals and they do not hurt. Before the test, the technician places the small electrodes on your head – the electrodes are held in place with a sticky paste. Th e electrodes are connected to the recording machine. Th e test lasts about 30 minutes and you will probably be sitting or lying down.

WHAT DOES AN EEG SHOW?

An EEG gives information about the electrical activity of the brain during the time the test is happening. When someone has an epileptic seizure their brain activity changes. This change can sometimes be seen on an EEG recording - it is often called epileptiform activity. Some people can have epileptiform activity even when they are not having a seizure, so an EEG can be particularly useful for them. Epileptiform activity can sometimes be provoked by deep breathing. The test may include deep breathing to see if epileptiform activity can be provoked and recorded.

YOUR RESULTS

An EEG test can usually show if someone is having a seizure at the time of the test, but it can't show what happens in the person's brain at any other time. So even though your test results might not show any unusual activity it does not rule out having epilepsy. Some types of epilepsy are very difficult to identify with an EEG test.

Some people who do not have epilepsy can sometimes have irregular activity on their EEG. But a result where there is irregular activity does not necessarily mean that the person has epilepsy.

FLASHING LIGHTS DURING THE EEG

Some people with epilepsy have seizures that are started, or 'triggered', by flashing lights. This is called photosensitive epilepsy and it affects up to 5% of people with epilepsy. An EEG test will usually include testing for photosensitive epilepsy. You will be asked to look at a light which will flash at different speeds. If this causes any changes in your brain activity the technician can stop the flashing light before a seizure develops.

SLEEP-DEPRIVED EEG

For some people there is more chance of irregular brain activity happening when they are tired or when they are going to sleep. If this is the case for you, having a sleepdeprived EEG might help get a more useful reading. This test is done in the same way as a normal EEG but you sleep during the test. To help you sleep, you may be asked to stay awake some, or all, of the night before. In some cases you may be given a mild sedative to help you get to sleep.

AMBULATORY EEG

An ambulatory EEG works in the same way as a normal EEG but is portable. It is a mall machine that is worn on a belt around your waist. Because it is portable you can move around and carry on with your normal day-to-day routine while the recording happens. This type of EEG allows brain activity to be recorded for several hours, days or weeks. Because the brain activity is recorded for longer, there is more chance of a seizure being recorded on the EEG than during the normal 30 minute test.

VIDEO TELEMETRY

Video telemetry testing happens in hospital, usually over a couple of days. During your stay you have your own room. In the room, often mounted on the wall, there is a video camera that records what you are doing. At the same time you will wear a portable EEG so that you are able to move around your room. Being videoed whilst wearing an EEG means that if you have a seizure your doctor can compare the electrical activity of your brain with what is happening to your body. Th e results can help identify what types of seizure you are having, and the most appropriate way of treating them.

BRAIN SCANS

Brain scans can be used to help fi nd the cause of someone's seizures. Th e scans produce pictures of the brain which might show a physical cause for epilepsy, such as scarring on the brain. But for many people a brain scan does not show up a cause for their seizures, and even if nothing unusual is seen, the person may still have epilepsy.

Th e two common types of brain scan are Magnetic Resonance Imaging and Computerised Axial Tomography.

MAGNETIC RESONANCE IMAGING (MRI SCAN)

An MRI scan uses strong magnetic fi elds to take images of the brain. Because of the magnetic fi elds, metal objects in or near the machine can aff ect, or be aff ected by, the machine. Before having an MRI scan you will need to remove any metal objects such as jewellery, hearing aids, coins or keys.

If you have a heart pacemaker or any surgical implant that contains metal you may not be able to have an MRI scan.

WHAT HAPPENS DURING AN MRI SCAN?

The scanner makes a loud noise so before it starts you will be given earplugs to wear. You will also be given a buzzer to hold - you can use the buzzer to let the technician know if you are feeling uncomfortable or unwell during the scan. The technician is usually on the other side of a window in another room during the scan, but an intercom means you can talk to them. There is also usually a mirror inside the scanner so you can see the technician during the scan. You may be able to have someone in the room with you during the scan.

During the scan you will lie on a platform which slides backwards into the scanner. When having an MRI scan to help diagnose epilepsy the scan usually takes about 30 minutes. Lying still during the scan is important so that the machine can take a clear image.

An MRI scan is usually a series of short scans with breaks in between rather than one long scan. Between each short scan the technician might use the intercom to check that you are comfortable. Computerised axial tomography (CT or CAT scan) CT scans use X-rays to take images of the brain. CT scans are not suitable if you are pregnant because the X-rays could affect an unborn baby. During a CT scan you lie on a couch which slides into the scanner.

CONFIRMED

Well around all of these diff erent medical tests everything still steamed in my head. Th is from the fact that doctors had no way and I had little way of controlling these tingling stomach sensations. Maybe it was a neurological problem but were these nerve cells in my stomach connecting to some part of my brain. Who knows!! Doctors would go back and forth: "We think it could be epilepsy but we are not sure." all saying and stating different things. By now I had been plastered with this Sodium Valporate 600mg of a morning and 1000mg at night.

I would, constantly have to be repeating everything. Th is as to what was going on about sudden jumping in the night. Whilst also all concerning these giggling sensations min my stomach. Plus also a red rash of which I was getting on the left side of my face. Of course "We will have to wait for the EEG results!" neurologists and doctors would constantly be saying to me.

But suddenly in 1986, at the age of fi fteen horror!! Because everything was confi rmed to me. At the Queen Aston Univercity at King Edward Vi House, 1 Aston Street Eastside, Birmingham B4 7ET. "We are sorry Lee, the EEG test results have just come through. "You are having nighttimes grand mal Epileptic seizures!" doctors told me.

This was terrible news!! So now I had epilepsy while also still getting these tingling sensations. What was all of this? I had started to suffer tiredness due to the medication. Plus occasional brief episodes of dizziness of which was really making my life fun!! Well what could I say do or think? Still at the Childrens Hospital seeing Dr J.D. Varley. But now I had also started seeing another neurologist named Dr. Tim Betts. Who worked at Aston Univercity in King Edward Vi House, 1 Aston Street Eastside of Birmingham. In the West Midlands of the United Kingdom.

Somehow I was starting to have around six tonic-clonic seizures whilst asleep a month. These of which I knew nothing about because I would be jumping in and out while sleeping. It was all quite confusing, so wondering what these forms of seizures were we had a chat with Dr J.D. Varley and Dr Tim Betts both in Birmingham.

They both told us all about different forms of epileptic seizures. "Tonic Clonic seizures and all the ones of which Lee is suffering with at night. "These are generalised seizures involving the whole brain. "It is the seizure type most people think of when they think of epilepsy. "Some people may experience an 'aura' such as a feeling of deja vu, a strange feeling in the stomach or a strange taste or smell, just before the seizure begins. "The aura itself is a simple partial seizure." Dr J Varley and Dr Tim Betts stated. Well eventually my family and I were to leave the Children's hospital of Ladywood. Next in the middle of 1986 it was time for regular tests and conversations about the epilepsy with neurologists. All at the

Queen Elizabeth Hospital in Edgbaston and now also Aston University of which are both in Birmingham.

I often visited Dr Tim Betts at the neurology department regularly as the epilepsy went on every day. Starting with what had sounded like simple partial attacks. With these tonic clonic seizures at night that were coming from the left temporal lobe of my brain. Th e tonic clonic seizures increased and became more frequent, so next I was put onto the tablet named lamotrigine.

POCKET MONEY

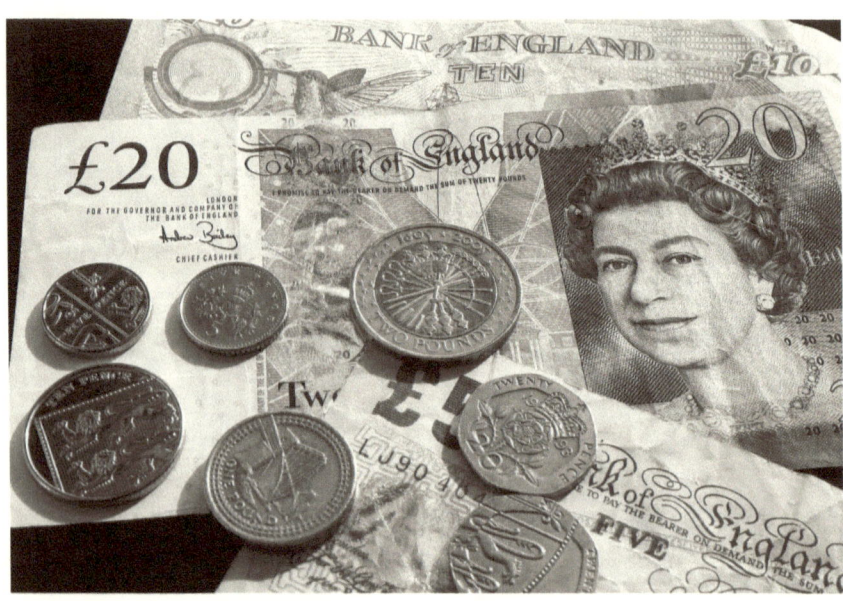

Well, even though I had this sudden shock of epilepsy. I still had good fun with mates as I went on everyday at Dartmouth High School. Everything was to be hard work but at the same time I made my school years a lot of fun. Because constantly as much as I studied. I was still one of the back row comedians in class. I would work hard in the English, Maths, Science and P.E. lessons. But sometimes in class I would be chucking paper direct at my teacher. Crack on! I thought. "Good shot, Lee!" my mates would say. Then "Who threw that!" the teacher shouted. Finding out it was me well then I would have to walk out. Th is to the front and apologise to my tutor and the class.

Eventually because of me throwing paper more than once, it was ruler time. "Whack!" across the hand and also sometimes I was to stand at the front of the class. Or even outside the room. I was still to eventually do well achieving many things. Because in my third year of school education. I started playing rugby in and outside of the school lessons. In sports lessons I would play for Churchill. While at other times playing for Dartmouth High School around Walsall and Birmingham. Th roughout this at school my tutor Les Cusworth. Who played rugby for Leicester and England found me a very good athlete and Rugby player. So off I went onto trial in rugby for a local West Midlands side named Hansworth.

Outside of that one good story was when going along to school with my Big D Bag. Or should I say: Big Dick bag, as my mates would call me. Th is bag was unbelievably a free present from my Grandad Geoff. He got it free from the Big D peanuts company. If anything cost my Grandad Geoff money he always made sure he got something back for it. I remember when I was a little boy, especially concerning my pocket money. I would go around to his off-licence and when asking him if I could have some sweets. Well "Yes you can Lee, have ten pence worth." So I got the sweets and put them into a paper bag. But suddenly "Lee, don't forget to put the ten pence in the till for your sweets." Grandad Geoff would say. On another occasion as I reached my late twenties. We were on our way up to the Albion soccer ground. We went past a side street store for hot dogs and burgers. Suddenly, "lee can you get me a burger, "Here is the pound to pay for the hamburger." But then of cause: "Lee, can I have the 1 pence change please." he said. I was laughing in shock it was crazy, because the burger cost 99 pence. It was unbelievable. But something though and that was even though he was stingy with money. Well he really cared and was always there to give me any help or advice about things.

WHY ME!

Still fun at school some of these were as mentioned, that I'm a huge fan of Roxy Music, collecting all of their albums and singles. In the year of 2005, I had the fantastic honour of meeting three of the group. Th ey were Phil Manzanera the guitar player, Paul Th ompson the drummer and Andy Mackay the saxophone player only Bryan Ferry of the group to meet all from Roxy Music. Th is had been one amazing dream. Along with two other groups that will be mentioned. Another interesting thing was in 1985. I had been watching the Live Aid concert show at London. Th ere were 1.4 billion television viewers worldwide glued watching this on the T.V screen. At the time of watching this I was living in another area of Birmingham named Sutton Coldfi eld.Th is was just down the road from Great Barr and just down the road from my school at the Scott Arms.

Th is day withLive Aid on the television it was really funny. Soon Bryan Ferry came onto the television I pressed the recording button straight away on the recorder to tape him singing four songs. He was to sing three songs from his new Boys and Girls album; "Sensation, Boys and Girls, Slave to love", then to fi nish his part of the show, "Jealous Guy," which was the number one hit single from Roxy Music in 1981.

Eventually of course, as many others around the world, (If not already there at Wembley,) just sang like myself all hearing loud and clear over their televisions and radios. Th is when suddenly all of the concert pop stars came out together at 21.56 to fi nish the concert by singing the song, "We are the World!" While the story caries on the main thing I write about. Th is is that I have so many joyful memories of school and when living in Birmingham. Along with music and soccer, another of my many interests would be collecting soccer programs.

I always went to second hand soccer program shops now having millions. Many of these shops were in Birmingham and West Bromwich. By then and looking now in my folders there are many of the F.A. Cup Final, League Cup and West Bromwich Albion programs. Th e soccer programs of Albion I have go back in many years gone past to around 1943. Many are worth a large amount of money now. Well now still I think in shock as I write in the story.

This about all that was to come. Even now in 2010, I get the memories inside my head. This of how have experienced so much. With thoughts of what could have often been the causes to have tingling sensations and this form of epilepsy in the years gone by. Will people ever understand how a person suff ers inside? I have suff ered dramatically hundreds of times daily. Why should people have to suff er? Just thought would it never stop. Psychologically your brain can play tricks with your mind. But luckily I was able to control mine. How I wanted to scream and shout out. **"Why me! Why me!"**

Everybody gets upset. But confidence and determination that would always enable me to live many unbelievable years to come.

Looking into the next few years there became many unbelievable situations many of which are to become very happy to remember throughout the year of 2011 often visiting would be made on going down to see Dr Mullatti at Kings College in London.

Having got up on this one special day became memories of the funeral to my Granddad Georges after passing away aged 91 sometime became spent down in the area of Droitwich at his funeral which was not so much happy but there are lots of him many occasions were made to seeing Granddad after experiencing a heart attack whilst he stayed in recovery at Stafford Hospital.

Regular occasions were made after changing to see him whilst looking and seeing to very much improve in Cannock Hospital something of which time became regularly made was Wednesday plus Sunday for weights plus running and aerobics in Stafford.

Everything here became arraigned and made in Staffordshire Leisure Centre for more occasions than needed three hours as well involving health often visits would be made going along to the Barbery seeing Dr Hugh Rickards in my home city of Birmingham.

Pleasure came at one night in which meeting people surrounding the football league became something special for everybody importance came along by seeing numerous politicians around England discussing health problems such as hospitals in Britain.

Suddenly arriving as was done into the National indoor Arena football became found involving many of the west midlands teams they were West Bromwich Albion plus Aston

Villa along with Birmingham City and others like Wolves and Walsall plus Coventry.

TABLE

Concentration as expected surrounding the year would obviously involve epilepsy and how my health came revolving the seizures often here the main concern became sudden eye twitching plus along with muscle stiffening and light spasms still aware of all disbelief arrived on the second occasion with Dr Rickards explaining that it looked as though epilepsy was nothing experienced by me.

Obviously the operation in 2007 had cured me but explain to him about the present experiences what was then being experienced suddenly fantastic!!! Because went along to see the football seeing Aston Villa 1 – 2 Albion in Villa Park on Saturday 22nd October.

Great Day gone as well in arriving!!! This became the first visit ever in seeing an international in the capital of London with many watching the match definitely produced interest finishing England 1 -0 Spain it certainly gave people something to remember well.

Pleasure came along when the telephone rang and on answering found out it became the BBC with Midlands Today news for wanted stories this became of which Ambulances plus hospitals are contacted so often for no reason and making stories on me proved we do need them.

Well something at the beginning just of expectation involving medical problems defiantly brought in regular exciting some unbelievable stories for this year going on into 2012 and this year certainly became something for remembering because of the experiences which came along regularly throughout the year coming.

As usual regularly contacting radio stations was constantly done discussing many things like football but often involving health care around all still unbelievably meetings were going along concerning Stafford hospital of which never seemed to be improving less education plus unclean hospitals.

Well this could have been explained by me often over the years surrounding personal visiting to hospitals one if not all of them in England now then along with constant exercise along plus around Stafford Leisure Centre had always been aerobics plus running and weights.

The big shock for something which came along later unbelievable in seeing became after buying two tickets from this company off the net bought for the European Championship Semi-final in Warsaw of Poland everything bought in those tickets came for £1284.00 confirmed.

Superb seeing the man worshiped because on the date of Saturday 26th May other tickets somewhere else came to see the greatest singer defiantly Axl Rose, yes!!! He became seen in the National Indoor Arena playing along with everybody else of Guns N Roses live he was fantastic.

So what came of them well this visit into see the family it was time for seeing different places along with our big football game in Warsaw.

Beginning this tour places going was made by setting off to see the European Championship football clubs in the polish capital.

Setting off by train was done first going along into Warsaw then once arriving it next became time for going on along for the football stadium

This was the Legia Warsaw ground with on arriving security was outside but extraordinarily on horses eventually the tickets were got.

Then it was time for excitement as on going inside the stadium it was pretty much like going along into Wembley voices and all soon began.

Unexpectedly whilst sitting with many Germans around 40,000 plus the same in Italians the sound of "Polska We Hate Germany!" heard in disbelief.

Well luckily this is not what had been sung it had been "Poland White and Red" the colours going into the Polish flag around the stadium.

Next on it was into looking around Glavitza plus Katovitza also including Krakow and Swierkland all cities in their country inside Poland.

Suddenly whilst in Glaviza it was heard and seen on television that my all time favourite were playing live in the city close to us whilst staying.

Well heard and going on down to Rybnik the personal all time singer Axl Rose was playing live along with his band worshiped by me.

Unbelievable when he started just like the other times having seen him live the voice was absolutely amazing listening along to them play!!

After the concert next as mentioned it was up to Krakow where there is an unbelievably massive shopping centre along with many pubs around.

Aura

Next day it became the returning back to England but with great memories like the European Semi-final plus seeing the group Guns N Roses live.

Next back home thoughts came of visiting the Olympics which became chosen having tickets to Earls Court and seeing Vollyball whist there.

Expectedly due to offers on the property the house was eventually brought off the Market on Thursday 4, April.

Interestingly something which always involves savings for people is having some ISA's with banks personally money became motivated along for that on Friday 5th April 2013.

Next it was off to see the result of Albion 2 – 1 Arsenal on Saturday 6th April when going along for the match in West Brom.

Soon it became the new match where it ended Albion 1 – 1 Newcastle in the great match to watch on Saturday 20th April.

Certainly funny as on Friday 26th whilst cutting the garden lawn it became mowing straight into the wire.

Next Saturday came along and the result on Saturday 4th, May ended Wigan 2 – 3 Albion good result for an away match.

Unexpectedly but known came on Sunday, 5th May when came along this seizure it became the worst one so far that year.

Here came Norwich v Albion for the away match on Sunday 12, May but the excitement certainly came as usual from 6.30.

This was the expected of once getting up next when dressed it became the 40 minute walk from one end unto the other.

By this meaning walk and sometimes run all the way to Stafford Leisure Centre when on arrival it became time for exercise.

Reaching there came an hour on the running machine and next came the joining of Dianne and the class of ladies for Aerobics.

Stupidity arrived on Tuesday 14th when time came for me to go up for Newcastle surrounding this new bus pass expected.

So the BIG soccer day arrived and my personal favourite ever because on Sunday 19th May came along this fantastic.

This was the match between West Bromwich Albion and Manchester United which ended up goals unbelievably through both.

Once reaching the end it finished Albion 5 – 5 Manchester United certainly goals for seeing as all finished great match.

Finished seeing it on Match of the day certainly helped me gather on regular as matches did how good the football that afternoon was.

Work came along when making along with one website company interest to my personally home webpage for epilepsy.

Having made it numerous people came on just making you realise sometimes how many people do go through this condition daily.

FIRST TIME ARRIVED!!! This became on Wednesday, 29th May seeing England 1 – 1 Republic of Ireland at Wembley never before.

The only misfortune became that Shane Long being this fantastic player scored for Ireland and his league team were the Albion.

Aura

Great first time with loads more to come in London at our international capital stadium of which England play in whenever playing.

Next but not new became constantly every night running up and down the Eccleshall Road on this occasion did two up and down.

Going in and around still brought on regular seizures Sunday 9th June four became experienced whilst trying to sleep in bed.

On regular occasion it would be such things like sharp eye twitching in the viewing or trying to sleep of different occasions constantly.

Plus with Seizures arriving suddenly as sleeping bad times would be if going into one awake because of the facial right hand side of my face twitching for 20 minutes or so but eventually slowing down and finishing.

Soon to arrive was the regular visit to Kings College to see Dr Mullatti getting there became some real mess from and through trains.

This was because after reaching Euston constant stopping and holding on came from them all due to rebuilding of the train station.

So instead of trains it ended up being this bus of which took us all over to hospital for this appointment at Kings and updating.

Soon as expected though became constant news everyday which has still not stopped today and this was complaints involving quality of hospitals.

John Kennedy

Knew it because suddenly 11 NHS hospitals have been given the reasons of poor care on special measures new this would come out eventually.

This could have been told to the government and general public by me along time in the past hospitals have always been poor quality.

Constant bad seizures would come along regularly easily up to the region sometimes on occasion they would still be coming around on floor.

If this was to happen then once coming around and standing up regularly there would and still is no knowledge as to where I am.

Saturday arrived and this brought along Albion 2 – 0 Bologna of which became played on Saturday 10th August for some more enjoyment.

Now this became the match not in forgetting because going along to see the next international certainly brought unexpected things.

Because even though being and supporting and the result ending England 3 – 2 Scotland somebody very important scored then what?

Forgot did I well yes and when James Morrison scored for Scotland it was jump up in celebration thinking there was this goal for the Albion.

Well of course he had scored for Scotland not the Albion in that international at Wembley luckily there became an explanation.

Sorry, telling everybody around me that even though he just scored for the opposition I supported West Brom as well like England.

Well along throughout medical problems regularly arriving with expectation but massive hopes of no more the bodily jerking still came.

Regular following of the Baggies has always brought along fun even though on Saturday 17th August we lost West Brom 0 – 1 Southampton.

As usual the next day would bring along time for getting up and going off to get exercise doing aerobics with girls in the class every time was fun.

Next would arrive to more matches one was to be played from the reserves on Friday 23rd August finishing Albion 0 – 3 Manchester United.

Soon it would be football and in the League Cup Round two finishing Albion 3 – 0 Newcastle on Tuesday 27th August for the next round.

Wembley, Wembley!!! Football again at this stadium viewing England 4 – 0 Moldova great for watching another great memory to see.

Expectations came as on Saturday 21st September the match finishing West Brom 3 – 0 Sunderland arrived great for seeing more memories.

Luckily but not successful came the League Cup 3rd Round where the result after 90 minutes finished Albion 1 – 1 Arsenal but so.

After that everything went into extra-time and after that still finishing the same along came penalties which finished Albion 4 – 5 Arsenal.

Well along came the big premier league match where the coach went up to Old Trafford in Manchester to see Man Utd 1 – 2 Albion was there.

Surrounding more days of exercise and plenty of work my health did not seem to be going through a bad patch which made me happy.

As regular arrival of football with plenty for seeing this as well being in need of supporting the team for my Grandad Geoff.

The match became much better even though still we got the point finishing Albion 1 – 1 Arsenal on Sunday 6th October maybe next time.

Soon though came international football again where it resulted England 4 – 1 Montenegro on Friday 11th October at Wembley.

Interesting experiences were to come again tomorrow as the coach was reached on the road for the trip down to London and not hospital.

Polska! Polska! Well on Tuesday 15th October came the very big match for qualifications of going in for World Cup 2014.

This meaning time was made and spent down for seeing England 2 – 0 Poland at Wembley superb game with the great atmosphere.

Next day gave the return journey for Stafford on what became loaded with people going back up along for the West Midlands we got three.

Now back the regular stories of life in the year at home so Howard his 65th birthday arrived for him this great footballer in the 1960 team.

Trained with many famous people had been at Lilleshall National Sports and Conferencing Centre along with receiving professionalism

By this am explaining that Howard played football for Shrewsbury Town becoming this fantastic footballer eventually to roll on into golf.

Soon to come along became more football as on Saturday 2nd November after the full week of work enjoyment along involving the gym.

Regular visiting plus having fun in aerobics or on bike racing plus weights and running became made as usual mostly Wednesdays and Sunday.

Of cause having supported the Baggies since 1977 more came on Saturday 2nd November finishing Albion 2 – 0 Crystal Palace that day.

Often appointments became made with people such as Jeremy Lefroe about regular daily subjects involving people in and surrounding England.

Excitement again because football even though the match resulting England 0 – 1 Germany on Tuesday 19th November still fun.

Earlier on in the day Windsor Castle had been visited having enjoyment in touring along throughout the building eventually returning.

By this meaning coming back on Wednesday 20th November all the way in National Express trains returning back to Stafford and going home.

Along it soon became time for going down for my appointment with Dr Mullatti on Friday, 22nd November returning to Kings in London.

Unfortunatly revolving around each day of disagreement or people becoming aggressive could well and did on Sunday 24th November into seizures.

These though as regularly experienced were different to epileptic being called Non-Epileptic seizures and on this date three were experienced.

Out from the mind and so came the big local derby between Villa and the Albion from 8.00pm on Monday 25th November ending in a 1 – 1 draw.

Still constantly exercise was to be made where at unbelievably three hours plus became regularly done in Stafford Leisure Centre this the next day.

Obviously returned every Sunday came still for the one hour special in aerobics doing well for all the ladies and people exercising around.

Beginning the last month of the year enabled plus time became made for designing then making Christmas cards for everybody throughout.

Obviously soccer still arrived where on Wednesday 4th December the Albion resulted losing 2 – 2 against Manchester City in the Hawthorns.

Next in line came Norwich but we lost on Saturday 7th December from them 0 – 2 at the Albion ground at 3.00pm unfortunately that day arriving.

Reaching the neuro-psychology department in Aunty Diannes car it time for seeing Dr Hugh Rickards the top neurologist of Birmingham.

Originally he was seeing me in teenage years whilst training along and working with Dr Tim Betts certainly one in top doctors for epilepsy.

Was anything done well being explained to me that staying on Kepra plus more would help reduce and control the seizures coming off could help.

In this meaning the less medication to be on would very much bring somebody very much more as me aware of all not so drugged up and slow.

Often thoughts are realised but unnoticed by the public in that if somebody is on any form of high dosage of tablet everything can really make them look slow.

That day was for seeing Dr Rickards nothing but discussion went on whilst having talked him in the region of 4.00pm there in the Queen Elizabeth Hospital.

Education again because the week earlier had become the start of an English lesson along with many in Stafford College studying of my old BTEC.

Having been in the class for exercise and "Zumba" soon it became time for Tom and me of going along to one very special party for Willie Johnson.

This all underwent at West Bromwich Albion football club on the evening of Thursday, 12th December meeting lots of famous football players whilst there.

Misfortune really hit me on the day at Friday, 13th December because health really became trouble having two long seizures plus one migraine.

Having written the first book named the "Magic Bullet!!! By Lee Rzepkowski many day had been spent going around Stafford to people about all.

Returning came the Baggies playing against but drawing with Hull City finishing 1 – 1 at home on Saturday 21st December in the Hawthorns again.

Eventually Christmas Day arrived so all became time for parties so the family got set up with each other for celebrations at Mum and Howard my dad their house.

John Kennedy

Soon came football again between the Albion and Tottenham Hotspher of London

Along came the eve of new year's day where time became spent along down at Stafford Leisure Centre for sure like usual just expected.

Well interesting year certainly many stories involving football of cause not forgetting those England International matches plus many other things along the line.

Did this Leap through university having studied and working on everything every day until well after 2.30am in the morning it was unbelievably found out that of doing to well of the health service course.

Interesting experiences arrive which come along regularly throughout every bodies life in plus around general plans surrounding life in and surrounding general experiences of the world constantly.

Supporting along with educating everybody has and will always be very important for the general whilst along with the government plus NHS this shall always be something needed for one to all in plus around.

Everything comes over free in England but quality in following the NHS sometimes might night be something flowed with as much quality in plus around hospitals along with doctors plus neurologists and more.

Defiantly something very useful and rare has been three operations to which have been undertaken by myself taking and achieving something being as serious like brain surgery unbelievably on three occasions.

Success has unbelievably improved this problem where on having auras surgery has reduced the strength unbelievably in plus throughout daily life since 2007 after undergoing the fourth operation in London.

Now then let me talk about something involving certainly involving personal interests of which has always been football since being taken along for seeing West Brom having just reached the age of eleven.

Some interesting results came along involving the Baggies when they beat teams such as Manchester United in Old Trafford one goal to nil plus many other matches have arrived throughout many days throughout the year plus expectedly going along supporting West Bromwich Albion either at home of their ground or expectedly places such as Wembley.

This stadium become more involved through watching England international matches

Whilst going along and watching the Albion came along by supporting them at places like Old Trafford home of Manchester United or Emirates Stadium along with may be the home of Arsenal in London

Plenty has been seen along and throughout experiences to discuss often in and throughout everybody revolving throughout unbelievable stories in as well surrounding the world.

Along the way exercise has constantly been of great importance with me to keep myself healthy going along for the gym has been of big importance whether in machine running or weights plus maybe doing something like Aerobics.

Many things arrive constantly throughout different seems in extraordinary situations bringing some fantastic information along each way has and always shall give important support to everybody of all throughout the world.

Wednesday31st December

Spent the day in the hotel on this evening soon Magda came over then eventually we both went out along to the parks to celebrate New Year's Eve at the parks.

Happy New Year!!!

On returning for the building

Thursday 1st January

Throughout the day stayed in plus around Glavitza along with everything time became spent relaxing for the night.

Friday 2nd January

Expectedly at this moment the hotel became left from Glavitza next in going along to Katavitza enabling me to come home flying back through Ryan Air into Birmingham International Airport were on arriving Mum plus Aunty Di and Tom picked me up from next driving me back to my flat at the Scott Arms of Great Barr in Birmingham then in all time just became relaxing for the night around.

Went along over to see the football match between the Baggies and Gateshead everything being run in the F.A. Cup 3rd round on Saturday 3rd January success defiantly arrived because the result ended us winning 7 – 0 involving them.

Expectedly which regularly happens with my personal superb General Practitioner Dr Aktar came along where time arrived for updating the health along at picking up medication and taking everything next for the chemist where tablets newly arrived like Epilm plus Kepra along with Lamotrage and Lacosamide involved to support my health.

2012

This year certainly became something for remembering because of the experiences which came along regularly throughout the year coming.

As usual regularly contacting radio stations was constantly done discussing many things like football but often involving health care around all.

Still unbelievably meetings were going along concerning Stafford hospital of which never seemed to be improving less education plus unclean hospitals.

Well this could have been explained by me often over the years surrounding personal visiting to hospitals one if not all of them in England.

Now then along with constant exercise along plus around Stafford Leisure Centre had always been aerobics plus running and weights.

The big shock for something which came along later unbelievable in seeing became after buying two tickets from this company off the net.

Bought for the European Championship Semi-final in Warsaw of Poland everything bought in those tickets came for £1284.00 confirmed.

Superb seeing the man worshiped because on the date of Saturday 26th May other tickets somewhere else came to see the greatest singer.

Defiantly Axl Rose, yes!!! He became seen in the National Indoor Arena playing along with everybody else of Guns N Roses live he was fantastic.

So what came of them well this visit into see the family it was time for seeing different places along with our big football game in Warsaw.

Beginning this tour places going was made by setting off to see the European Championship football clubs in the polish capital.

Setting off by train was done first going along into Warsaw then once arriving it next became time for going on along for the football stadium

This was the Legia Warsaw ground with on arriving security was outside but extraordinarily on horses eventually the tickets were got.

Then it was time for excitement as on going inside the stadium it was pretty much like going along into Wembley voices and all soon began.

Unexpectedly whilst sitting with many Germans around 40,000 plus the same in Italians the sound of "Polska We Hate Germany!" heard in disbelief.

Well luckily this is not what had been sung it had been "Poland White and Red" the colours going into the Polish flag around the stadium.

Next on it was into looking around Glavitza plus Katovitza also including Krakow and Swierkland all cities in their country inside Poland.

Suddenly whilst in Glaviza it was heard and seen on television that my all time favourite were playing live in the city close to us whilst staying.

Well heard and going on down to Rybnik the personal all time singer Axl Rose was playing live along with his band worshiped by me.

Unbelievable when he started just like the other times having seen him live the voice was absolutely amazing listening along to them play!!

After the concert next as mentioned it was up to Krakow where there is an unbelievably massive shopping centre along with many pubs around.

Next day it became the returning back to England but with great memories like the European Semi-final plus seeing the group Guns N Roses live.

Next back home thoughts came of visiting the Olympics which became chosen having tickets to Earls Court and seeing Vollyball whist there.

2013

Thursday 4, April 2013

Expectedly due to offers on the property the house was eventually brought off the Market on Thursday 4, April.

Interestingly something which always involves savings for people is having some ISA's with banks personally money became motivated along for that on Friday 5th April 2013.

Next it was off to see the result of Albion 2 – 1 Arsenal on Saturday 6th April when going along for the match in West Brom.

Soon it became the new match where it ended Albion 1 – 1 Newcastle in the great match to watch on Saturday 20th April.

Certainly funny as on Friday 26th whilst cutting the garden lawn it became mowing straight into the wire.

Next Saturday came along and the result on Saturday 4th, May ended Wigan 2 – 3 Albion good result for an away match.

Unexpectedly but known came on Sunday, 5th May when came along this seizure it became the worst one so far that year.

Here came Norwich v Albion for the away match on Sunday 12, May but the excitement certainly came as usual from 6.30.

This was the expected of once getting up next when dressed it became the 40 minute walk from one end unto the other.

By this meaning walk and sometimes run all the way to Stafford Leisure Centre when on arrival it became time for exercise.

Reaching there came an hour on the running machine and next came the joining of Dianne and the class of ladies for Aerobics.

Stupidity arrived on Tuesday 14th when time came for me to go up for Newcastle surrounding this new bus pass expected.

So the BIG soccer day arrived and my personal favourite ever because on Sunday 19th May came along this fantastic.

This was the match between West Bromwich Albion and Manchester United which ended up goals unbelievably through both.

Once reaching the end it finished Albion 5 – 5 Manchester United certainly goals for seeing as all finished great match.

Finished seeing it on Match of the day certainly helped me gather on regular as matches did how good the football that afternoon was.

Work came along when making along with one website company interest to my personally home webpage for epilepsy.

Having made it numerous people came on just making you realise sometimes how many people do go through this condition daily.

FIRST TIME ARRIVED!!! This became on Wednesday, 29th May seeing England 1 – 1 Republic of Ireland at Wembley never before.

The only misfortune became that Shane Long being this fantastic player scored for Ireland and his league team were the Albion.

Great first time with loads more to come in London at our international capital stadium of which England play in whenever playing.

Next but not new became constantly every night running up and down the Eccleshall Road on this occasion did two up and down.

Going in and around still brought on regular seizures Sunday 9th June four became experienced whilst trying to sleep in bed.

On regular occasion it would be such things like sharp eye twitching in the viewing or trying to sleep of different occasions constantly.

Plus with Seizures arriving suddenly as sleeping bad times would be if going into one awake because of the facial right hand side of my face twitching for 20 minutes or so but eventually slowing down and finishing.

Soon to arrive was the regular visit to Kings College to see Dr Mullatti getting there became some real mess from and through trains.

This was because after reaching Euston constant stopping and holding on came from them all due to rebuilding of the train station.

So instead of trains it ended up being this bus of which took us all over to hospital for this appointment at Kings and updating.

Soon as expected though became constant news everyday which has still not stopped today and this was complaints involving quality of hospitals.

Knew it because suddenly 11 NHS hospitals have been given the reasons of poor care on special measures new this would come out eventually.

This could have been told to the government and general public by me along time in the past hospitals have always been poor quality.

Constant bad seizures would come along regularly easily up to the region sometimes on occasion they would still be coming around on floor.

If this was to happen then once coming around and standing up regularly there would and still is no knowledge as to where I am.

Saturday arrived and this brought along Albion 2 – 0 Bologna of which became played on Saturday 10th August for some more enjoyment.

Now this became the match not in forgetting because going along to see the next international certainly brought unexpected things.

Because even though being and supporting and the result ending England 3 – 2 Scotland somebody very important scored then what?

Forgot did I well yes and when James Morrison scored for Scotland it was jump up in celebration thinking there was this goal for the Albion.

Well of course he had scored for Scotland not the Albion in that international at Wembley luckily there became an explanation.

Sorry, telling everybody around me that even though he just scored for the opposition I supported West Brom as well like England.

Well along throughout medical problems regularly arriving with expectation but massive hopes of no more the bodily jerking still came.

Regular following of the Baggies has always brought along fun even though on Saturday 17th August we lost West Brom 0 – 1 Southampton.

As usual the next day would bring along time for getting up and going off to get exercise doing aerobics with girls in the class every time was fun.

Next would arrive to more matches one was to be played from the reserves on Friday 23rd August finishing Albion 0 – 3 Manchester United.

Soon it would be football and in the League Cup Round two finishing Albion 3 – 0 Newcastle on Tuesday 27th August for the next round.

Wembley, Wembley!!! Football again at this stadium viewing England 4 – 0 Moldova great for watching another great memory to see.

Expectations came as on Saturday 21st September the match finishing West Brom 3 – 0 Sunderland arrived great for seeing more memories.

Luckily but not successful came the League Cup 3rd Round where the result after 90 minutes finished Albion 1 – 1 Arsenal but so.

After that everything went into extra-time and after that still finishing the same along came penalties which finished Albion 4 – 5 Arsenal.

Well along came the big premier league match where the coach went up to Old Trafford in Manchester to see Man Utd 1 – 2 Albion was there.

Surrounding more days of exercise and plenty of work my health did not seem to be going through a bad patch which made me happy.

As regular arrival of football with plenty for seeing this as well being in need of supporting the team for my Grandad Geoff.

The match became much better even though still we got the point finishing Albion 1 – 1 Arsenal on Sunday 6th October maybe next time.

Soon though came international football again where it resulted England 4 – 1 Montenegro on Friday 11th October at Wembley.

Interesting experiences were to come again tomorrow as the coach was reached on the road for the trip down to London and not hospital.

Polska! Polska! Well on Tuesday 15th October came the very big match for qualifications of going in for World Cup 2014.

This meaning time was made and spent down for seeing England 2 – 0 Poland at Wembley superb game with the great atmosphere.

Next day gave the return journey for Stafford on what became loaded with people going back up along for the West Midlands we got three.

Now back the regular stories of life in the year at home so Howard his 65th birthday arrived for him this great footballer in the 1960 team.

Trained with many famous people had been at Lilleshall National Sports and Conferencing Centre along with receiving professionalism

By this am explaining that Howard played football for Shrewsbury Town becoming this fantastic footballer eventually to roll on into golf.

Soon to come along became more football as on Saturday 2nd November after the full week of work enjoyment along involving the gym.

Regular visiting plus having fun in aerobics or on bike racing plus weights and running became made as usual mostly Wednesdays and Sunday.

Of cause having supported the Baggies since 1977 more came on Saturday 2nd November finishing Albion 2 – 0 Crystal Palace that day.

Often appointments became made with people such as Jeremy Lefroe about regular daily subjects involving people in and surrounding England.

Excitement again because football even though the match resulting England 0 – 1 Germany on Tuesday 19th November still fun.

Earlier on in the day Windsor Castle had been visited having enjoyment in touring along throughout the building eventually returning.

By this meaning coming back on Wednesday 20th November all the way in National Express trains returning back to Stafford and going home.

Along it soon became time for going down for my appointment with Dr Mullatti on Friday, 22nd November returning to Kings in London.

Unfortunatly revolving around each day of disagreement or people becoming aggressive could well and did on Sunday 24th November into seizures.

These though as regularly experienced were different to epileptic being called Non-Epileptic seizures and on this date three were experienced.

Out from the mind and so came the big local derby between Villa and the Albion from 8.00pm on Monday 25th November ending in a 1 – 1 draw.

Still constantly exercise was to be made where at unbelievably three hours plus became regularly done in Stafford Leisure Centre this the next day.

Obviously returned every Sunday came still for the one hour special in aerobics doing well for all the ladies and people exercising around.

Beginning the last month of the year enabled plus time became made for designing then making Christmas cards for everybody throughout.

Obviously soccer still arrived where on Wednesday 4th December the Albion resulted losing 2 – 2 against Manchester City in the Hawthorns.

Next in line came Norwich but we lost on Saturday 7th December from them 0 – 2 at the Albion ground at 3.00pm unfortunately that day arriving.

Aura

Reaching the neuro-psychology department in Aunty Diannes car it time for seeing Dr Hugh Rickards the top neurologist of Birmingham.

Originally he was seeing me in teenage years whilst training along and working with Dr Tim Betts certainly one in top doctors for epilepsy.

Was anything done well being explained to me that staying on Kepra plus more would help reduce and control the seizures coming off could help.

In this meaning the less medication to be on would very much bring somebody very much more as me aware of all not so drugged up and slow.

Often thoughts are realised but unnoticed by the public in that if somebody is on any form of high dosage of tablet everything can really make them look slow.

That day was for seeing Dr Rickards nothing but discussion went on whilst having talked him in the region of 4.00pm there in the Queen Elizabeth Hospital.

Education again because the week earlier had become the start of an English lesson along with many in Stafford College studying of my old BTEC.

Having been in the class for exercise and "Zumba" soon it became time for Tom and me of going along to one very special party for Willie Johnson.

This all underwent at West Bromwich Albion football club on the evening of Thursday, 12th December meeting lots of famous football players whilst there.

Misfortune really hit me on the day at Friday, 13th December because health really became trouble having two long seizures plus one migraine.

Having written the first book named the "Magic Bullet!!! By Lee Rzepkowski many day had been spent going around Stafford to people about all.

Returning came the Baggies playing against but drawing with Hull City finishing 1 – 1 at home on Saturday 21st December in the Hawthorns again.

Eventually Christmas Day arrived so all became time for parties so the family got set up with each other for celebrations at Mum and Howard my dad their house.

Soon came football again between the Albion and Tottenham Hotspher of London

Along came the eve of new years day where time became spent along down at Stafford Leisure Centre for sure like usual just expected.

Well interesting year certainly many stories involving football of cause not forgetting those England International matches plus many other things along the line.

Thursday 4, April 2013

Expectedly due to offers on the property, the house was eventually brought off the Market on Thursday 4, April.

Interestingly something which always involves savings for people is having some ISA's with banks personally money became motivated along for that on Friday 5th April 2013.

Next it was off to see the result of Albion 2 – 1 Arsenal on Saturday 6th April when going along for the match in West Brom.

Soon it became the new match where it ended Albion 1 – 1 Newcastle in the great match to watch on Saturday 20th April.

Aura

Certainly funny as on Friday 26th whilst cutting the garden lawn it became mowing straight into the wire.

Next Saturday came along and the result on Saturday 4th, May ended Wigan 2 – 3 Albion good result for an away match.

Unexpectedly but known came on Sunday, 5th May when came along this seizure it became the worst one so far that year.

Here came Norwich v Albion for the away match on Sunday 12, May but the excitement certainly came as usual from 6.30.

This was the expected of once getting up next when dressed it became the 40 minute walk from one end unto the other.

By this meaning walk and sometimes run all the way to Stafford Leisure Centre when on arrival it became time for exercise.

Reaching there came an hour on the running machine and next came the joining of Dianne and the class of ladies for Aerobics.

Stupidity arrived on Tuesday 14th when time came for me to go up for Newcastle surrounding this new bus pass expected.

So the BIG soccer day arrived and my personal favourite ever because on Sunday 19th May came along this fantastic.

This was the match between West Bromwich Albion and Manchester United which ended up goals unbelievably through both.

Once reaching the end it finished Albion 5 – 5 Manchester United certainly goals for seeing as all finished great match.

Finished seeing it on Match of the day certainly helped me gather on regular as matches did how good the football that afternoon was.

Work came along when making along with one website company interest to my personally home webpage for epilepsy.

Having made it numerous people came on just making you realise sometimes how many people do go through this condition daily.

FIRST TIME ARRIVED!!! This became on Wednesday, 29th May seeing England 1 – 1 Republic of Ireland at Wembley never before.

The only misfortune became that Shane Long being this fantastic player scored for Ireland and his league team were the Albion.

Great first time with loads more to come in London at our international capital stadium of which England play in whenever playing.

Next but not new became constantly every night running up and down the Eccleshall Road on this occasion did two up and down.

Going in and around still brought on regular seizures Sunday 9th June four became experienced whilst trying to sleep in bed.

On regular occasion it would be such things like sharp eye twitching in the viewing or trying to sleep of different occasions constantly.

Plus with Seizures arriving suddenly as sleeping bad times would be if going into one awake because of the facial right hand side of my face twitching for 20 minutes or so but eventually slowing down and finishing.

Soon to arrive was the regular visit to Kings College to see Dr Mullatti getting there became some real mess from and through trains.

Aura

This was because after reaching Euston constant stopping and holding on came from them all due to rebuilding of the train station.

So instead of trains it ended up being this bus of which took us all over to hospital for this appointment at Kings and updating.

Soon as expected though became constant news everyday which has still not stopped today and this was complaints involving quality of hospitals.

Knew it because suddenly 11 NHS hospitals have been given the reasons of poor care on special measures new this would come out eventually.

This could have been told to the government and general public by me along time in the past hospitals have always been poor quality.

Constant bad seizures would come along regularly easily up to the region sometimes on occasion they would still be coming around on floor.

If this was to happen then once coming around and standing up regularly there would and still is no knowledge as to where I am.

Saturday arrived and this brought along Albion 2 – 0 Bologna of which became played on Saturday 10th August for some more enjoyment.

Now this became the match not in forgetting because going along to see the next international certainly brought unexpected things.

Because even though being and supporting and the result ending England 3 – 2 Scotland somebody very important scored then what?

Forgot did I well yes and when James Morrison scored for Scotland it was jump up in celebration thinking there was this goal for the Albion.

Well of course he had scored for Scotland not the Albion in that international at Wembley luckily there became an explanation.

Sorry, telling everybody around me that even though he just scored for the opposition I supported West Brom as well like England.

Well along throughout medical problems regularly arriving with expectation but massive hopes of no more the bodily jerking still came.

Regular following of the Baggies has always brought along fun even though on Saturday 17th August we lost West Brom 0 – 1 Southampton.

As usual the next day would bring along time for getting up and going off to get exercise doing aerobics with girls in the class every time was fun.

Next would arrive to more matches one was to be played from the reserves on Friday 23rd August finishing Albion 0 – 3 Manchester United.

Soon it would be football and in the League Cup Round two finishing Albion 3 – 0 Newcastle on Tuesday 27th August for the next round.

Wembley, Wembley!!! Football again at this stadium viewing England 4 – 0 Moldova great for watching another great memory to see.

Expectations came as on Saturday 21st September the match finishing West Brom 3 – 0 Sunderland arrived great for seeing more memories.

Luckily but not successful came the League Cup 3rd Round where the result after 90 minutes finished Albion 1 – 1 Arsenal but so.

After that everything went into extra-time and after that still finishing the same along came penalties which finished Albion 4 – 5 Arsenal.

Well along came the big premier league match where the coach went up to Old Trafford in Manchester to see Man Utd 1 – 2 Albion was there.

Surrounding more days of exercise and plenty of work my health did not seem to be going through a bad patch which made me happy.

As regular arrival of football with plenty for seeing this as well being in need of supporting the team for my Grandad Geoff.

The match became much better even though still we got the point finishing Albion 1 – 1 Arsenal on Sunday 6th October maybe next time.

Soon though came international football again where it resulted England 4 – 1 Montenegro on Friday 11th October at Wembley.

Interesting experiences were to come again tomorrow as the coach was reached on the road for the trip down to London and not hospital.

Polska! Polska! Well on Tuesday 15th October came the very big match for qualifications of going in for World Cup 2014.

This meaning time was made and spent down for seeing England 2 – 0 Poland at Wembley superb game with the great atmosphere.

Next day gave the return journey for Stafford on what became loaded with people going back up along for the West Midlands we got three.

Now back the regular stories of life in the year at home so Howard his 65th birthday arrived for him this great footballer in the 1960 team.

Trained with many famous people had been at Lilleshall National Sports and Conferencing Centre along with receiving professionalism

By this am explaining that Howard played football for Shrewsbury Town becoming this fantastic footballer eventually to roll on into golf.

Soon to come along became more football as on Saturday 2nd November after the full week of work enjoyment along involving the gym.

Regular visiting plus having fun in aerobics or on bike racing plus weights and running became made as usual mostly Wednesdays and Sunday.

Of cause having supported the Baggies since 1977 more came on Saturday 2nd November finishing Albion 2 – 0 Crystal Palace that day.

Often appointments became made with people such as Jeremy Lefroe about regular daily subjects involving people in and surrounding England.

Excitement again because football even though the match resulting England 0 – 1 Germany on Tuesday 19th November still fun.

Earlier on in the day Windsor Castle had been visited having enjoyment in touring along throughout the building eventually returning.

Aura

By this meaning coming back on Wednesday 20th November all the way in National Express trains returning back to Stafford and going home.

Along it soon became time for going down for my appointment with Dr Mullatti on Friday, 22nd November returning to Kings in London.

Unfortunatly revolving around each day of disagreement or people becoming aggressive could well and did on Sunday 24th November into seizures.

These though as regularly experienced were different to epileptic being called Non-Epileptic seizures and on this date three were experienced.

Out from the mind and so came the big local derby between Villa and the Albion from 8.00pm on Monday 25th November ending in a 1 – 1 draw.

Still constantly exercise was to be made where at unbelievably three hours plus became regularly done in Stafford Leisure Centre this the next day.

Obviously returned every Sunday came still for the one hour special in aerobics doing well for all the ladies and people exercising around.

Beginning the last month of the year enabled plus time became made for designing then making Christmas cards for everybody throughout.

Obviously soccer still arrived where on Wednesday 4th December the Albion resulted losing 2 – 2 against Manchester City in the Hawthorns.

Next in line came Norwich but we lost on Saturday 7th December from them 0 – 2 at the Albion ground at 3.00pm unfortunately that day arriving.

Reaching the neuro-psychology department in Aunty Diannes car it time for seeing Dr Hugh Rickards the top neurologist of Birmingham.

Originally he was seeing me in teenage years whilst training along and working with Dr Tim Betts certainly one in top doctors for epilepsy.

Was anything done well being explained to me that staying on Kepra plus more would help reduce and control the seizures coming off could help.

In this meaning the less medication to be on would very much bring somebody very much more as me aware of all not so drugged up and slow.

Often thoughts are realised but unnoticed by the public in that if somebody is on any form of high dosage of tablet everything can really make them look slow.

That day was for seeing Dr Rickards nothing but discussion went on whilst having talked him in the region of 4.00pm there in the Queen Elizabeth Hospital.

Education again because the week earlier had become the start of an English lesson along with many in Stafford College studying of my old BTEC.

Having been in the class for exercise and "Zumba" soon it became time for Tom and me of going along to one very special party for Willie Johnson.

This all underwent at West Bromwich Albion football club on the evening of Thursday, 12th December meeting lots of famous football players whilst there.

Misfortune really hit me on the day at Friday, 13th December because health really became trouble having two long seizures plus one migraine.

Having written the first book named the "Magic Bullet!!! By Lee Rzepkowski many day had been spent going around Stafford to people about all.

Returning came the Baggies playing against but drawing with Hull City finishing 1 – 1 at home on Saturday 21st December in the Hawthorns again.

Eventually Christmas Day arrived so all became time for parties so the family got set up with each other for celebrations at Mum and Howard my dad their house.

Soon came football again between the Albion and Tottenham Hotspher of London

Along came the eve of new year's day where time became spent along down at Stafford Leisure Centre for sure like usual just expected.

Well interesting year certainly many stories involving football of cause not forgetting those England International matches plus many other things along the line.

NHS HOSPITALS

Around all of this though visiting hospitals has always been of regular importance for me there have pluses areal many experiences which come along explained one way or the other about health care reform improvements involving epilepsy for me regularly beneficial changes have arrived helping destinations to arrive provincially for one and all surrounding life in and revolving the world but even though the health service at Kings in London are praised by me there is also plenty unbelievable.

Because so much could have been explained many years ago revolved which NHS hospitals must be defiantly the worst form of buildings and service ever invented surrounding the world defiantly since the year of July 5 1948 at its start has been one very lucky form of help but having personally been in so many it has seemed terrible because the rooms are dreadfully built and looked after those have independently been seen around the time personally since the date of my life.

Even though let us begin with an unbelievable story to somebodies personal life which on reading if living in England will not surprise you but defiantly by living outside of the country shall expectedly confuse you defiantly after personally hearing how good the Health Service has been in places for instance like the American hospitals which are looked after so well everything for helping one plus all here is terrible.

Next shall we explain then, regular confusion in room taking comes as well here situations like medication arrive being incorrect qualification as well just regularly realised but not straight away throughout with personality disorders often by NHS workers is disgraceful every day it could have been explained like done to Mum about the personal treatment given unbelievably having machines plus needles inserted into my head Electrodes and many more sockets bringing unbelievable pain by explaining not everybody has been amazing some but very few have been poor luckily for me.

Let us begin the story by voice what has defiantly been something on telling people has never been heard of in form anywhere else in England because it will shock you in certainty because on this certain date was to change everything for certainly the new future enabling so much achieved to be discussed enabling loads unbelievably to arrive from myself since life arrived in and out every day to something else not gathered.

Extraordinarily sometimes we never understand the most important needs in life for some reason many health problems have and probably will never be understood which does not enable the government at having installing plus supporting anybody with health concerns in many very little sometimes as well in any way surrounded in our times luck has been very good to me along with paramedics in ambulances of all.

Throughout England here we receive something name our National Health Service as mentioned of which became available to everybody on the 5 July 1948 but since then even though many improvements have come along support and financial help involving people with something called "Mental Health" problems very few words should not ever be used by people myself the general house of Commons has just spent 50 Million on medical problems should more be spent.

Looking around hospitals can regularly be quite shocking for the quality and support offered inside which is personally noticed through past and present visits to many over the country on most occasions in the capital plus the second top city known of my home country that shows how much needs to be rebuilt along with learning inside for all as mentioned but it has become only that the house of commons has only spent 50 million on the health service in England.

Now then visiting places such as the Guys Maudsley hospital of which has and still is unbelievably out in date plus having been the place of which two very serious personal operations were under taken once in teenage years with electrodes inserted into the scull like some doll and then next in 1992 the place in which the personal first operation came to me has plus now is used for MRI Scanning enabling medical people in seeing the damage if any concerning the brain unfortunately mine has been on the left side in surrounding my brain.

COMPLAINING

Along with every electrode being moved results took ages with ideas personally of nothing so complaints plus telephone conversations were constantly made but as explained then being told of not having epilepsy what had my personal doctor been on about when discussing everything with me one thing became discussed which became Non-Epileptic seizures of which shall be discussed later in the story as knowledge from any plus probably everybody in general ether have no education or very little surrounding differences revolving epileptic plus the other seizures just mentioned surrounding and unfortunately being experienced by myself today.

Disbelief came whilst having electrodes on this sudden experience because whilst having the electrodes inserted onto my head on this occasion whilst sitting on the bed one with many more were taken out but experiencing so much education had been terrible for one nurse because she nailed one electrode back into my head which really hurt so next personally after that getting up off the bed and taking the electrode box along with any electricity and went for complaining about her from the occasion that fifty electrodes had been inserted into the head and next staying for confirmation and all in Kings afterwards everything really started in complaints.

Returning became time for speaking to PALS or Patient and Liaison Supporters group which are involved in any complaints of anytime surrounding any if not all hospitals around Britain because if anybody causes trouble in any of all medical and NHS buildings then by contacting these people they shall report everything over to every hospital of which it was experiences next everybody involved shall become in trouble and even on occasion if ever something becomes bad then whoever shall be sacked why has education plus machinery always been poor for neurology like this.

SAFETY

Gathered with those we still have different machines involving the NHS buildings at which look around in plus outside really unbelievably out from date for surrounding timed walls are damp the floors are only concrete with appositely no carpet just like what became viewed inside the hollies in 2015 when seeing little Natalie it really has been dreadful the way general are looked after in NHS buildings with so few concrete floors not painted or clean and unsafe beds.

Rooms where tests are undertaken really need updating even the machinery in whatever form has and still is dreadful this could have been explained from me on the first visit in the 1970's surly the government can see by going throughout and looking in surrounding the produced which basically in view every NHS bed plus building shows mistreatment of patients terrible.

Memories bring in stories daily involving Stafford hospital concerning elderly care plus cleanliness of rooms and the building itself became unbelievable plus having been the place which on many occasions has been visited by me do to becoming poorly another person that spent some time in that hospital became my Granddad George Grice after becoming poorly the health service in general have been superb in my eyes it has always been medical buildings which are constantly poor memories come over from Dr Hannigan my G.P in Stafford well his general surgery looked like some back garage hospitals along with the English medical service really has got some bad name presently the new one for me now is this man again another great General Practitioner at home.

Still though after being interviewed on BBC News this was reported for the television on 26 August 2014 the story became discussed about West Midlands Ambulance Service being called 661 times to one Birmingham general public at home.

Ambulances were called to one Birmingham home 661 times but only 12 callouts led to hospital visits.

West Midlands Ambulance Service released details of the 10 top 999 callers in a year and the number of times people went to hospital.

BBC Midlands Today also discovered 396 callouts to a Newcastle-under-Lyme home, leading to 77 hospital visits.

Where people had "complex health-related disorders" calls were "entirely appropriate", said the service.

"The trust is aware of a number of high-volume service users who sometimes call the ambulance service every day or more," said a service spokesman.

"Some people do suffer from complex health-related disorders that at times require emergency intervention on a regular basis and although this may appear to be a 'misuse' of resources it is indeed entirely appropriate."

Lee Biddle, who suffered up to eight epileptic seizures each day from the age of 17, said he could not say whether the number of callouts to any address was high as he said "it depended on the condition".

Mr Biddle said: "If you see someone unconscious, it's obvious you've got to help that person. If you don't know how to put someone in an epileptic seizure the right way around, the ambulance has got to be called."

Robert Cole, the service's head of clinical practice, said it worked to put in place care packages so individuals had an alternative to calling ambulances frequently.

They could include agreeing a plan for an individual's ongoing treatment with their GP or involving other agencies to help people who had complex mental health disorders, he said.

He said the service was managing three categories of callers including those with complex health needs who genuinely needed an ambulance and those with complex needs who did not. He said there were also vexatious callers who might call to ask "to turn the heating down, let the dog outside or to water the plants". Became the full story.

Still inside medical wards though people are constantly trolled around like some food rolled deal in superstores where the surrounded beds are automatically being terrible plus in explanation along with food discussed is no better tasting dreadfully worse memorising misfortune like of plenty more everything from school food understanding plus improvement really is needed financially even though as discussed just earlier which is the English government have used 50 million for mental health problems but new hospitals make everybody plus their opinion just like mine terrible basically like jail plus involvement surrounding education inside such working properly can always be needed personally remember very well one experience where electrode needles shall and have been so painful.

SAFETY

Another memory has and shall always be whilst going through the hallway for surgery this one person was lying on this rock hard hospital bed and falling off obviously from notice going into some form of epileptic seizure care on that day seemed dreadful how can people not take view or care for somebody becoming so poorly this just about shows how out from date the NHS buildings plus on regularity subliming education for one and all in for everything surrounding our services of England.

OPINIONS

Personal thoughts come along with major praise for NHS workers that have been involved this myself because every time on going along for hospital who ever becomes gathered in the subject next it will always be added and still does come along with helpful workers plus ideas for coming on in to improve my health whether involving medication or more with the National Health Service.

Even though being trolled in and out from hall ways then into rooms as walls are just as poor as the floors unpainted plus not clean beds nearly as hard like the floor along with no security from any accidents like somebody experiencing an epileptic seizure then they can collapse onto the rock hard floor from the bed with nothing but electrical wires from such things as plugs and testing machines falling on them.

VIEWED

Walking into any medical building looks the same from top unto bottom as the ground floor plus stairs come along revolving hall ways onto hall ways looking and becoming as rock hard from concrete as any other white paint coming off walls from everywhere coffee expensive with tables and chairs falling to pieces with anything from coffee plus other drinks like tea being expensive along with homemade food tasting as bad as school food something remembered also is the state where some concrete floors have broken misplacing concrete pieces involving many places in and reviewing these buildings in all.

This can be dreadful because often wheel Chairs are disgraceful in make and use when somebody can be dropped into some very tight cardinal metal chair then stormed around throughout hallways in surrounding different wards television screens dreadfully out from date in plus throughout rooms whether computerised for EEG tests or maybe heart plus many other forms of tests along with surgery anywhere needing repair.

ELECTRICAL

Wires as mentioned can be left all over floors from not only alarms plus CCTV footage but screen monitors obviously to many machines by doors along with also hall ways which can not only just cause damage to electric cords but more trouble for patients and visitors walking in and outside of the rooms unbelievably disbelief arrives when being the patient because on many beds you are caged up.

Many of these home comforts have the metal sidings hanging off causing many with epilepsy and other conditions to either fall out or bang their heads on by the line something else are metal doors might be something witnessed with doors hanging off some with graffiti on also windows show nothing and are metaled up not enabling people to look through unless with some form of magnifying glass because there is nothing

In the corner of rooms also most are not clean because you see bits of rubbish and dust around every ward plus room is like some jail cell and so poorly kept plus often elevators do not work many beds are left outside plus unclean from rooms where many can have no entry on the doors due to cleaning or repainting other things might be telephones of which need to be used shall be broken and hanging off walls everywhere.

Bricks might arrive jumping out in front of you another can and has been the capital of Kings College hospital involving here just off Denmark Hill Drive station near Euston on the verge by the stop taking about forty minutes from the capital train station outside and reverting near for the stop which surrounds many places involving loads of long straight roads surrounding the capital of London in the United Kingdom will and should change everything in and surrounding NHS Hospitals.

OTHER DEPARTMENTS

Pharmacies and receptions are so unbelievably kept often there are nobody to help somebody on arriving to speak about appointments plus for need to help at directions for rooms and wards eventually causing people to be late for meetings unbelievably places of need for medication along with forms involving tablets can be hidden away like tents often having not tablets either.

What is deeply studied today well something called Non-Epileptic seizures which are the main objectives connected with myself and defiantly something which certainly brings no understanding into life are problems these Non-Epileptic Seizures most experienced through general people but with somebody being aggressive with the person already having epilepsy these look just the same as epileptic seizures but misfortunate people having the problem actually feels the same the general do not knowing of when they are going into one normal or Non-Epileptic seizures.

Confusion and misunderstanding will so often bring the incorrect formation into people for life many terrible accusations which reiterate problems twice as bad by injunctions defusing objectives regularly make anything certainly to which puts aggression into stress certainly will cause neurology to deteriorate and misunderstanding often epilepsy.

What personally happens is the body stiffens then pressure arrives into the left arm next causing the collapsing of and jerking onto the floor then suddenly whilst hearing all which is going on around the body this person has no control whilst eyes are closed and the body unluckily ends up on the ground looking unconscious for quite some time of it.

What are they and how is this form of condition made needing treatment plus help with little understanding by medical if not all people however in and around the places of life much need of discussion along with understanding is something needed enabling everybody to communicate more things and disabilities which all people go through unintentionally throughout life in plus involving the world.

2014

Unbelievable confidence along with determination has taken me along way where there have not only been experiences of surgery but also visiting to places around the world like America meeting loads of general as well like many people meeting us everybody has a story to tell but some of these very few have to explain in this form do you know anybody that has undergone surgery of some form it can be really difficult but anybody having this has to be very strong which is defiantly something involved in my personality.

As mentioned in the next book we shall talk about loads of superb experiences like different sports such as the New York Giants much more on the Kennedy family in one way or another we shall discuss everything for you to enjoy thinking he like this story so much has been achieved but these are very happy forms of enjoyment to discuss.

Life can look so enjoyable and now living in Birmingham surrounded with a little girl plus wife and dog defiantly brings times to remain and getting back to Great Barr certainly has been an achievement in itself of which was hoped in since childhood my little daughter Natalie looks identical to me and is healthy whilst all of my family live in Stafford plus friends around the world make the most because there is and shall be unbelievable things for everybody like you to achieve so hope you enjoyed reading the story and look forward for the next life shall get even better for as mentioned yourself along with everybody around life and the world but many forms of tests and then the only person to have undergone brain surgery four times confidence goes along way.

Lee.

www.ingramcontent.com/pod-product-compliance
Lightning Source LLC
Chambersburg PA
CBHW030839180526
45163CB00004B/1381